WITH

Praise for the 7pm to 7am Sleeping Baby Routine

'To the mother and father of the baby who is not sleeping, I know how it can feel, having been in the situation three times myself. There are solutions and this book explains them in a succinct way, drawing on real science. Charmian's practical advice deals with many of the common gut problems that babies experience, such as lactose intolerance, cow's milk protein allergy and reflux. You discover ways to ensure your baby is happier and more comfortable so that you can get a good night's sleep. I would endorse it fully and wholeheartedly.'

– Professor Mike Thomson, Professor of Paediatric Gastroenterology at The Portland Hospital, London

About the author

Charmian Mead is a highly successful newborn sleep, routine and breast-feeding consultant who has been teaching her method for 20 years. She started her career in childcare as a nanny 27 years ago and has since worked all over the United Kingdom and internationally, helping parents to establish routines and consulting on a range of baby-related issues. During her years working with new parents, she has developed a sure-fire way of helping babies to sleep through the night from a very early age.

A note from the author

My unique method for helping babies to get a full night's sleep is based on decades of experience working with babies and children. As you will see, at times my approach differs from general government advice in the UK. Throughout the book, I will explain how my method differs from current government recommendations and offer compromises, so that you can make your own decision about what is best for you and your child. For further guidance on my methods, see the video tutorials on my website: www.sleepingbabyroutine.co.uk.

7pm to 7am
Sleeping Baby
Routine

7pm to 7am
Sleeping Baby Routine

The no-cry plan to help your baby sleep through the night

CHARMIAN MEAD
The Baby Sleep Expert

Vermilion
LONDON

1 3 5 7 9 10 8 6 4 2

Vermilion, an imprint of Ebury Publishing,
20 Vauxhall Bridge Road,
London SW1V 2SA

Vermilion is part of the Penguin Random House group of companies
whose addresses can be found at global.penguinrandomhouse.com

Penguin
Random House
UK

First published by Vermilion in 2018

www.penguin.co.uk

A CIP catalogue record for this book is available from the British Library

ISBN 9781785041761

Typeset in 10.5/14.1pt Sabon LT Std
by Integra Software Services Pvt. Ltd, Pondicherry

Printed and bound by Clays, St Ives PLC

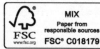

Penguin Random House is committed to a
sustainable future for our business, our readers
and our planet. This book is made from Forest
Stewardship Council® certified paper.

Contents

Acknowledgements

My friends and family, and most of the families I have worked with over the last 20 years, will know that this book has been a long time coming, but it is finally here!

Thank you to all the families I have worked with, who have put their trust in me with their most precious possession and who have allowed me to share and guide them through such a special time in their lives. It's been emotional and the most fun, even at four in the morning! Helping you all has also allowed me to live out my strong maternal instinct. Thank you to those families who have allowed me to use photos of their experiences as a guide for the illustrations in this book.

A special thank you to Chelly Reynolds and my father, Roger Mead, who have both helped with my inability to use a computer or Word properly and have been a constant, huge support with putting my book together.

I would also like to thank my aunt, Caroline Rees, for her early input with the structure of the book.

Lastly, I would like to dedicate this book to all the mummies out there, including my late mother Helena Mead.

Introduction

With over 25 years' experience working with babies and children, my passion has led me to become a successful newborn sleep, routine and breastfeeding expert, which has allowed me to help parents get a great start with their newborns. I have helped parents all over the United Kingdom and internationally. I decided to write this book to offer anxious, tired parents an alternative to sleepless nights and inflexible, 'one-size-fits-all' routines.

Many mothers I've helped over the years have remarked that it's a shame their little bundle of joy doesn't come with a user manual. (That, and an air valve for easy winding!) Clearly this is the result of a lack of planning on the part of the design department! The first three months with your baby, although exciting, can be a very emotional and exhausting time. This has not always been helped by health professionals, experts and other books on baby care offering advice that babies should be fed 'whenever they show signs of hunger' and considering it normal for a baby to wake several times a night. A few weeks of continual, frequent night waking can leave even the most resilient parent frazzled. It's quite likely that you are reading this book because you, like so many other parents, are sleep-deprived and unable to decipher your new arrival. Perhaps your baby is having feeding or digestive issues. Or maybe she is unable to self-settle to sleep and wakes frequently during naps and at night.

In today's baby world, there are generally two main schools of thought: the baby-led, feed on demand, co-sleeping approach versus the strict routine, controlled

1

crying method. I have been teaching my routine for 20 years now and, with my hands-on experience, I believe there is an urgent need for a more balanced, 'best of both worlds' approach. The *7pm to 7am Sleeping Baby Routine* focuses on your baby's digestion and an understanding of how to meet her every need. A baby's digestive comfort has an impact on how settled and relaxed she is, her ability to feed properly, sleep, stay awake and generally be happy in herself. My routine also teaches positive associations, for example sucking for food instead of for comfort or as an aid to falling asleep; self-settling instead of being rocked and cuddled to sleep; and learning the difference between night and day early on. My routine also encourages skin-on-skin cuddle naps as well as stimulating play.

The *7pm to 7am Sleeping Baby Routine* can be followed from birth or introduced at a later stage if you need help after weeks, or even months, of night waking. For those of you reading this book before the birth, or in the first couple of weeks afterwards, you will be able to start as you mean to go on – it's much easier to establish good feeding and sleeping habits now, at the start of your baby's life, than to break bad habits later on. And, by following the Sleeping Baby Routine, you could have your baby sleeping through the night for up to 12 hours as early as 6–8 weeks of age. How much of my routine you follow is up to you but, even if you apply just some of my '12 Steps for 12 Hours' Sleep' (page 153), it will have a positive impact and you will have a greater understanding of your new baby.

Why Me?

My maternal instinct has driven my passion and my routine is based on over 25 years of experience helping hundreds of babies sleep at night, mothers successfully breastfeed and families adapt to a routine within an already busy family life.

My routine has a newborn's needs, well-being and digestive comfort at the heart of it and the results speak for themselves: babies on the Sleeping Baby Routine are happy and thriving, sleep through the night from an early age, and quickly learn the difference between night and day.

My method is based on decades of experience and, as you will see, at times goes against general government advice. Throughout the book I will explain my methodology and offer compromises as well as outlining the current government recommendations so you can make your own decision on what is best for your child.

Why a Routine?

We all live our lives by routine. Many of us get up in the morning, have breakfast, go to work, and eat lunch and dinner at around the same time each day. Routines help us to feel secure, and it's no different for infants. For most babies who are fed on demand – the baby-led approach – the lack of structure means that they are essentially sorting out their own routine. As a result, your baby may well decide to sleep all day and be awake through the night, sleep while she is feeding or want to feed when you want her to sleep.

On a routine your baby will demand feeding every 3–4 hours, and often go longer between feeds during the day if left to her own accord. However, you will want to take advantage of these longer periods between feeds during the night so often you will need to wake your baby for her daytime feeds. In the first 6–8 weeks, if you feed your baby until she is naturally full, as my routine suggests, she will not need or want to be fed more frequently. You are not leaving your baby hungry, crying or waiting for feeds. If your baby is hungry, she is fed. You are merely making sure your baby feeds well and is wind-free at each feed period, encouraging some structured awake time to allow for digestion and to teach her the difference between night and day.

The advice to feed your baby whenever she shows signs of hunger – 'on demand' – means you could be reading your baby incorrectly as babies show signs of hunger, known as 'rooting', when they are hungry, but also when they are uncomfortable with wind and when they are tired. Interestingly, the advice for twins and multiple births is to routine feed your babies, even when these babies are often born at a much lower birth weight. So why would a routine be so controversial for a single baby? I believe the lack of NHS funding has had an impact on the advice given to new parents these days. It used to be that a mother stayed in hospital and was taught baby care and breast-feeding skills and now, with inconsistent advice, mothers are barely taught how to latch their babies to the breast and told to let their baby feed whenever she wants. With a routine that works the proof is in the results: a thriving baby who is gaining weight, sleeps well and has happy, calm playtime.

In my view, the first stage of parenting is to teach your baby to sleep at night. I am not totally against feeding babies 'on demand', but if you feed your baby until she is full, wind her regularly and structure awake time at each day feed, rather than giving short, frequent feeds of 5–10 minutes, she will *demand* her meals every 3–4 hours and fall into a natural routine.

The idea is to encourage, not to enforce, a routine. Babies are individuals with their own personalities and capabilities so don't expect your baby to act like a robot that can be pro-grammed. The Sleeping Baby Routine is based on structured days and baby-led nights offering a balanced approach with no controlled crying. Your baby will naturally sleep through the night at her own pace and this will become a habit that stays with her throughout childhood. Sometimes the routine will go like clockwork; sometimes it won't. When this happens, don't despair – I will show you options to adjust the routine accordingly, and always remember that tomorrow is another day! You can use my routine either as a broad guideline for a satisfied, happy baby or as a recommendation to be followed closely, so that your baby sleeps through the night much more quickly than is generally thought possible.

Think of the first six weeks of your newborn's life as 'establishing'. You are establishing a routine which will help you successfully breast- or bottle-feed, help your baby to thrive, teach her the difference between night and day, help her to sleep through the night and learn positive associations with eating, settling and sleeping. It can take the whole of the newborn stage – up to 12 weeks – to become established. The Sleeping Baby Routine will continue until your baby is weaned (at 4–6 months) and therefore needs to evolve, and be tweaked and adapted to your baby's individual behaviour and needs. Once you enter the baby phase, from three months onwards, you and your baby have become established. Whether she is in a routine or not, this is what your baby knows and is familiar with and she is now fully aware of her surroundings.

A few weeks into my routine and you should be able to see how the routine is working for you and your baby. Everyone will have an opinion on how you raise your child and you will hear a lot of conflicting advice. How you want to tackle the first three months, routine or no routine, is up to you. There is no right or wrong way. Advice is all that is given and you need to choose the right path for your own family.

Flexibility

Adults usually sleep for 7–9 hours per night, while babies and young children need 10–13 hours. The Sleeping Baby Routine is based on a 12-hour night and a 12-hour day. However, in the routines throughout this book I show the timings for a day that starts at 7am and ends at 7.30pm. This is because the bedtime routine often takes longer to establish during the newborn stage. Bedtime will probably get nearer to 7pm as you and your baby get used to the routine, and your baby becomes more efficient at feeding, her gut strengthens and she becomes self-winding. The Sleeping Baby Routine offers flexibility during the day – I have suggested variations of feed timings throughout so you can adjust the routine to fit with your family's lifestyle or your developing baby's needs – with baby-led nights and no controlled crying. Unlike 'traditional' routines, your baby does not need to be woken during the night for a 'dream feed', but is instead allowed to wake of her own accord.

Starting a routine from birth will mean you have some restrictions until you are established: a newborn is unable to stay awake while in motion; she is unable to wind herself; her gut is immature and needs to strengthen; and breastfeeding needs to be established. However, once you are out of the newborn stage, your routine will become less restrictive and structured. Feeds are efficient and quick, expressing takes 5–10 minutes, if needed, instead of 10–20 minutes, and winding becomes less frequent as your baby's gut strengthens. You'll find that, in time, your baby can take more milk between winding breaks, is able to self-wind and can easily stay awake during motion. It may feel like hard work for the first 4–6 weeks – it's a bit like learning to drive a car with so much to think about and do – but soon everything speeds up and becomes automatic.

The *7pm to 7am Sleeping Baby Routine* is a no-cry, common-sense guide. The end result is a happy, thriving baby who sleeps through the night on a very flexible routine.

Chapter One

The Gut: Wind and Digestive Issues

Your baby is born with a very small, immature gut and for some babies this is a sensitive zone which needs to be handled with care. The Sleeping Baby Routine focuses on your baby's digestion and works by gradually increasing his milk intake at each feed during the day to encourage sleeping at night.

Wind

Trapped air or burps (wind) that have not been released during and after feeds will have a marked impact on the quantity of milk your baby takes, how wakeful he is during playtime and how well he naps, not to mention the duration of sleep during the night. Wind gives your baby a false sense of fullness which can make him very sleepy initially, but then often causes vomiting as the air gets stuck behind the milk and pushes it out on the way up, resulting in a loss of milk intake. This can cause hunger and therefore disrupted sleep. Trapped wind can also cause pain as the air travels through your baby's immature digestive system and passes out the other end.

Babies are unable to wind themselves for the first 8–12 weeks of life. It's therefore important to wind your baby frequently – every 5–10 minutes on the breast or every 15–30ml

(½–1oz) on the bottle, or if he is falling asleep and comfort sucking – for the first six weeks. This is key to the success of my routine. As your baby's digestive system strengthens, he will be able to take more milk between burps, resulting in quicker feeds, reduced wind and less need for winding, and will be able to self-wind by 12 weeks. If your milk is very fast-flowing and your baby has a strong suck then break every two minutes for the first two or three winding breaks on each breast as the foremilk especially is lighter and more wind-forming. If your baby takes too much milk in the first feeding session before winding it can create a build-up of air that's hard to shift.

The winding process can get harder at Weeks 4–6 as the quantity of milk your baby takes increases dramatically in this time (your baby will have a growth spurt during this period), but then it starts to get easier again from Week 8. By this time, as your baby's appetite has slowed, he will have, in my experience, reached his maximum intake of milk per feed during the day, give or take a few ounces.

> *Myth: Breastfed babies do not need winding*
>
> Oh yes they do! And sometimes more so than bottle-fed babies, depending on Mum's diet. The foremilk especially is more wind-forming.

How to wind your baby

An ineffective winding technique is the most common cause of many of the problems that I come across. Here's what to do ...

Firstly, make sure the room is cool (19–20°C) and that your baby is feeding in a vest bodysuit only, not fully clothed and snuggly warm. It is important that your baby is wide awake before you start to wind him – it's near impossible to wind a sleeping baby. If your baby is sleeping, put him on a muslin on the floor and tickle him awake.

Sit your baby on your knee with one of your hands supporting his stomach up to the chest so he has a nice straight back. Newborns have undeveloped stomach muscles and are therefore unable to hold themselves up for the first 8–12 weeks, so you will need to lift your baby's diaphragm and support his stomach and chest into a sitting position, with your forefinger and thumb supporting his chin and head. Apply a little pressure to the stomach if he is tricky to wind. Pat his back with your other hand, cupping and moulding your hand around his back. By moulding your hand you are not directly patting his spine but either side of it. Rub his back using firm, circular, upward strokes. I often find that babies are being winded too gently and are often stroked to sleep rather than helped to bring the wind up.

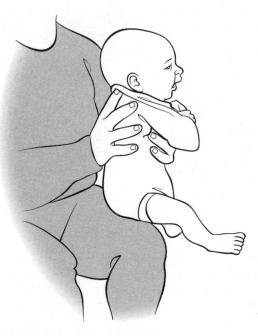

Winding your baby on the knee

Another effective winding position is over your shoulder:

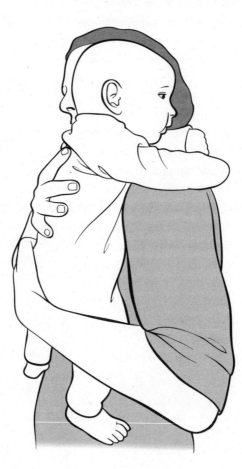

Winding your baby over the shoulder (also the best position for calming your baby)

However, if you have a sleepy baby this position is not recommended, as he will tend to fall asleep – the over-the-shoulder position is often a calming position used to stop crying and before bed to relax (see page 206 for more on this).

When winding your baby have a muslin at the ready as the burp will probably come with a posset too! Once your baby has released a good burp, put him back on the breast or bottle. Don't expect to hear tiny 'baby' burps – a baby can burp as loudly as an adult. Newborns often grunt and make throaty noises; don't mistake these for a burp. If your baby is passing wind frequently you are not getting all the air up during a feed.

Posseting versus vomiting

Recognising the difference between a posset, or throw up, and a proper sick or projectile vomit is important. Some babies will posset constantly throughout the day and others only while they are being winded or during feed periods. With most newborns I care for, I place a muslin under their head wherever they lie, be it in a Moses basket or on a play mat. A posset can be up to 7ml (¼oz). (If you are not sure what this amount looks like, try putting the equivalent quantity of milk in a washing up bowl to get an idea.) This amount is not worth re-feeding and is not a cause for concern – it's most likely due to wind.

Projectile vomiting or sicking up in excess of 30ml (1oz) is a proper vomit and you will need to re-feed the amount lost. Again, this isn't a cause for concern as babies are often sick – your baby is not ill. (A sick newborn is very rare – signs of illness to look out for are: vomiting after every feed, an inability to keep any milk down, your baby looking limp and lifeless, and/or a fever.) Babies are not sick like adults. The milk slides up and out easily without causing discomfort, unless, of course, it comes out of their nose. Only then will it shock, sting and upset your baby. Babies can projectile vomit their whole feed in one go, which is quite something to see and can be very alarming for new parents.

When your baby is being sick, keep him straight up in the seated, winding position and hold him there until he has finished. If sick does come through his nose, and he is upset by this, do not wipe his face until he is calm. Moving your baby while he is actually being sick and wiping him up before he has finished being sick can cause more milk to come up.

If your baby falls asleep during winding or it is taking a while to get the wind up, lay him on the floor, on a muslin, for a short time and tickle him awake – tickling his feet and the chest area can be particularly effective. Laying your baby flat can help shift the air bubble, but don't lie him down for more than a minute or so as this technique works so well with some babies that they can bring their milk back up.

Working out your baby's winding pattern can take time – does he regularly have one big belly burp or does he let out two or three smaller ones before he is able to feed again? Be patient when getting to know your baby. In time you will know exactly what is right for him.

As well as frequent, correct winding, you might want to add a daily dose of probiotics to your baby's feed to reduce the amount of wind he produces. High-strength probiotic powder added to one feed a day helps strengthen and balance your baby's gut and boost his immune system. Probiotic powder is the first port of call when I encounter babies with digestive issues, but I advise this for every baby, regardless of wind complications. If you are breastfeeding, try adding it to your baby's bedtime bottle. I use BioCare Baby BioFlora powder and add ¼ of a teaspoon to the bedtime bottle.

Causes of wind

A baby's drinking action – his sucking action and subsequent swallowing – is the usual cause of wind. The wrong sucking action or the wrong teat size or shape can cause excess wind. If you are bottle-feeding, you may need to experiment with different teats. If the milk is flowing too fast, it may spill out of your baby's mouth and he will have to gulp so fast that he takes on air too. If it is too slow, he has to suck hard for little reward, except a tummy full of air. The teat should fit well in your baby's mouth with no gaps at the side. In my opinion, the MAM teats are the best shape. (See page 102 for more information on the best bottle and teat to use.)

Some babies seem more prone to wind than others and there are several other possible reasons for this:

1. *Feeding in a flat position.* When breastfeeding, make sure your baby's head is higher than his feet and that his body is turned towards you so he is not feeding with his head turned to the side. When bottle-feeding, ensure that your baby's head is higher than his feet and his back is well supported.

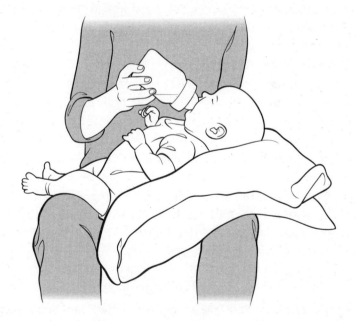

Ideal position for bottle-feeding

2. *Feeding too frequently.* If your baby is breastfeeding and 'snacking' – feeding too often or not for long enough and therefore never reaching the hindmilk – he could be taking too much foremilk. Foremilk is thinner and much windier than hindmilk or formula. Follow my routine to space out your feeds. Whether you are breast- or bottle-feeding, it is important to space out your baby's feeds to allow his stomach to empty before feeding again. Fresh milk on top of undigested milk with too frequent feeding creates a build-up of gas.

3. *Comfort sucking on the nipple/teat without drinking.* Most babies, given half the chance, will snooze and comfort suck, just happy to have something to half-suck on and have a cuddle. However, when your baby comfort sucks he loses focus and doesn't actually drink but uses the breast or teat as a comforter, much like a dummy.

4. *Tongue tie.* Tongue tie can cause digestive issues due to an ineffective suck and an inability to circular breathe while feeding, which makes for erratic feeding, gulping or comfort sucking. A baby with tongue tie will suck well for a minute or so but then the tongue falls back, and the baby loses energy and starts comfort sucking.

5. *A temporary gut sensitivity.* Gut issues tend to rear their heads at around Weeks 3–6 and get increasingly problematic. As your baby's gut strengthens, wind issues should decrease not increase after six weeks of age. Digestive issues, such as lactose intolerance, a cow's milk protein allergy, silent reflux, acid reflux and projectile vomiting, are all treatable once given the right diagnosis. My routine works with digestive issues making them easier to deal with given that the focus of my routine is the gut.

6. *Mother's diet when breastfeeding.* Wind-causing foods which lead to pain while digesting include: anything related to the onion and chilli family (this includes peppers and leeks), windy veg (such as cabbage, cauliflower and cucumber), spices, pulses and beans. These foods create

wind and add fuel to the fire of a windy tum. Pre-made foods, such as soups and sauces, are almost certainly made with onions, so make sure you always read the labels.

Digestive Issues Uncovered

Did you notice in the list above that there is no mention of the term 'colic'? I don't use this term because colic isn't a condition … Colic is a term used to cover a host of undiagnosed baby digestive issues. People throw this term around when they cannot explain or diagnose why a baby is in discomfort or upset. I've been teaching parents my routine for 20 years now and I have never had a baby in discomfort where I couldn't pinpoint the actual cause. A newborn's behaviour is based around the gut and it is important to look at your baby as a whole to find the cause of his symptoms. Unless a baby has a genuine gut issue, the usual reason for unexplained crying is, once again, hunger, a build-up of gas or not enough structured awake time during the day. So let's unravel the mystery around the term 'colic' and uncover the true possible reasons for your baby's upset.

Symptom: Long periods of crying or being unsettled from late afternoon to well into the evening, generally at the same time each day

Cause: A build-up of wind

If a baby is not winded thoroughly during feeds throughout the day a build-up of gas occurs after several feeds. This can be exacerbated by feeding too frequently where fresh milk on top of undigested milk in the stomach can cause wind and pain. It can take three hours for a baby's stomach to empty, depending on his milk intake.

Winding your baby regularly during feeds to stop the build-up of wind is so important for his comfort (see page 7 for guidance on this). It's common for newborns to have some kind of wind issues as they're unable to self-wind until 8–12 weeks old. If you are breastfeeding it's important to consider what you eat (see page 33).

Cause: Hunger due to a low milk supply

Often babies become more unsettled towards the afternoon and evening resulting in 'cluster feeding' (when babies feed regularly at certain times of the day). Mum thinks her baby is constantly feeding, when in fact the supply just isn't there and the baby is getting very little milk. It may look like your baby is drinking, but he may be comfort sucking and getting very little milk. Comfort sucking looks like a short up-and-down action, often with a shuddery jaw – nibble, nibble, pause, or a long pause with the occasional suck. In contrast, an active suck looks like a wide circular action with visible swallowing. When the milk supply has run out, the sucking action alone can pacify a baby like a dummy which sends him off to sleep, only for him to wake soon after because he is still hungry.

A mother's milk supply depletes throughout the day, in some cases dramatically from the afternoon onwards. Underestimating how much your baby needs to drink at any one feed will leave him hungry, especially towards the evening time. In theory, your milk supply is at its best in the morning as, having slept at night, your body has had a chance to rest and produce milk. Conversely, your milk supply is generally at its lowest in the late afternoon to evening, and this is when your baby needs his heaviest feed to set him up for the night ahead to encourage longer sleep periods overnight.

To combat this, my routine encourages you to express milk after the first two morning feeds and give expressed breast milk or formula in a top-up bottle before bed (see pages 58 and 171 for more on this). Expressing will encourage a good milk supply, which can take weeks to establish. Do be aware that it's common for some women to never produce enough milk to satisfy their baby's appetite, in which case night feeds will take much longer to phase out. In this case I would recommend mixed feeding (combining breastfeeding with bottle-feeding) to ensure your baby sleeps through the night (see Chapter Six for guidance on this).

Keep your baby awake and actively sucking during each feed for maximum breast stimulation and ensure you wind your baby thoroughly. Allowing some awake time after each daytime feed will help you to understand how much milk your baby is getting and whether he is full or not. If your baby is still looking hungry after an hour of feeding (unsettled straight after feeds or chewing on his hands), is not content during playtime and won't settle for his naps then you almost certainly have a low milk supply or your baby may not have drained your breasts due to falling asleep or comfort sucking. To help increase your supply, eat well between feeds, have skin-on-skin naps with your baby, go to bed early, eat between each feed, drink plenty of water and regularly express after the morning feed to stimulate your milk production. See page 29 for more advice on increasing your milk supply.

Symptom: Crying when put down to sleep

Cause: Not enough awake time, still hungry or unable to self-settle

Your baby may not be getting enough awake time during the day which can result in catnapping or an inability to settle himself. Some babies are born able to stay awake for two hours at a time, while others struggle to stay awake past a feed. Managing your baby's awake time and encouraging visual stimulation during the day will make for a peaceful night. Instinct tells us to put a baby down for a nap straight after a feed, as he becomes sleepy on the breast or bottle, but common sense says that this is the best time for him to be awake as, having a full tummy, he will be happy to look around and play.

This playtime will also give your baby an opportunity to digest his milk and alleviate any wind created while digesting. Try to increase your baby's awake time by 10–15 minutes over the first few weeks until he is able to stay awake for two hours at each feed period (this is an essential part of my routine) by 4–6 weeks of age. Try not to rock your baby or use other props to send him to sleep as these will only cause long-term issues with settling and sleeping (see pages 164 and 176 for more on this).

Teaching self-settling

Are you trying to help your baby settle to sleep? Rocking your baby to sleep and then transferring him to a Moses basket, pram or cot means that he is likely to wake while being transferred as he is no longer being rocked or cuddled on your chest. He may also wake soon after you put him down as the environment that he fell asleep in has changed. As your baby becomes more aware of his surroundings over the coming weeks this will be enough to disrupt sleep. Sleep aids, such as white noise and dummies, have a temporary settling effect, but will make a rod for your own back long-term as your baby will be unable to settle himself. It is therefore much kinder to start as you mean to go on and teach positive associations with settling and sleep.

Make sure your baby is getting enough milk at each feed. Ensure he is winded well and has had happy awake time after each daytime feed. These variables must be met in order for your baby to sleep. After playtime spend 10 minutes calming him down and having cuddles, but try not to let him fall asleep on you. If your baby is wakeful then swaddle him before a cuddle and then tuck him into bed so he feels secure while he settles and while he is asleep. Use the 'shush and hold' technique (see page 205) to help settle him if necessary.

Symptom: Crying during feeds and not settling between feeds

Cause: Flow issues or low milk supply

Again, this could be due to a low milk supply, which will only frustrate your baby as his appetite is not being satisfied. See page 29 for advice on how to increase your supply.

Crying during feeds and being unsettled between feeds could also be a result of not being winded enough during feeds or the flow of the teat or breast being too fast or too slow. A fast milk flow means your baby can gulp milk and take in excessive amounts of air and drink too much milk too quickly. The foremilk especially can be very fast-flowing. To combat this, express the first ounce from each breast before starting each feed. Wind your baby more frequently, ideally every two minutes for the first two or three wind breaks on each side. Rest assured that fast-flowing milk will be a blessing when your baby is slightly older and is able to self-wind, but it can be problematic for newborns.

If you are bottle-feeding, use a size one teat and wind your baby after every 15–30ml (½–1oz).

Cause: Acid reflux

The dreaded acid reflux is a common condition – affecting 1–5 per cent of babies – and is where a baby's stomach brings back strong gut acid as he starts to digest milk, which causes pain and discomfort while feeding. Symptoms of acid reflux start from a third of the way into the bottle or breastfeed once the milk has hit the baby's stomach, causing pain during digestion. Symptoms may include: excess wind and bloating, screaming and crying during the feed, and projectile vomiting due to trapped wind. The condition usually creeps in gradually at around 3–6 weeks of age as your baby increases his milk intake. Giving a course of probiotics is the first port of call which helps balance the gut and boost your baby's immune system (see page 12), but if the condition gets worse I would advise seeking out a specialist who will be able to prescribe medication for complicated reflux, such as an acid blocker like omeprazole, or an antacid like ranitidine.

The advice commonly given by GPs for babies with acid reflux is to feed your baby more frequently. I have cared for babies with reflux for 20 years and following my routine, which allows the baby's stomach to completely empty between feeds, causes less pain overall in a 24-hour period. Switching to a non-dairy diet, if you are breastfeeding, or to a lactose- or dairy-free formula, if you are bottle-feeding, may help with digestion and lessen the aggravation of symptoms.

Cause: Cow's milk protein (CMP) allergy or lactose intolerance

CMP allergy or sensitivity – a reaction to a protein found in breast milk (when the mother consumes dairy produce) and formula – is a common problem, with about 5 per cent of infants being affected. CMP allergy can last up until 10–12 months of age. Symptoms include:

- excess wind
- bloating
- pain while digesting
- loose stools
- mucus
- diarrhoea
- fussy feeding
- blood in stools

If your baby seems to be suffering from the symptoms of CMP allergy and you are breastfeeding, try eating a dairy-free diet or switch to a non-dairy formula milk if you are bottle-feeding.

Lactose intolerance is also a common problem for new-borns and causes pain during and after feeds, excess gas and sometimes vomiting. Try switching to a lactose-free formula if your baby appears to be suffering and a dairy-free diet if you are breastfeeding. Lactose intolerance gets worse towards Month 3 when the lactase enzyme is at its lowest level in the gut.

Symptoms of the two conditions are similar, so it can take some investigating to determine. Lactose intolerance is caused by an inability to break down lactose, the sugar found in milk and other dairy products, while CMP allergy is a food allergy caused by an allergic reaction to the protein in milk.

Your baby should be at his happiest when he is feeding. If this is not the case and your baby is crying and upset during feeds then something is wrong. If none of the advice I've given above helps your issue, you'll need to see your GP and your baby may be referred to a specialist to check whether he has a sensitivity or allergy.

Symptom: Crying during feeds and immediately after

Cause: Hunger or wind

If your baby is crying during or after a feed, it may be because he has trapped wind. Try winding your baby more frequently, making sure you are getting the burps up and out. Hunger is also another cause of a baby crying after a feed. If you suspect that your baby is still hungry, try increasing his milk intake by increasing your milk supply (see page 29) or by topping up with a bottle after the breastfeed (see page 70). If you are bottle-feeding, try gradually increasing your baby's milk intake by 30ml (1oz) at a time until the problem is solved.

Encouraging active sucking while feeding (see page 36) and allowing awake time after your baby's feeds will help you to understand if he needs more milk and is wind-free.

Dummies

I am not a fan of dummy use! In my experience, dummies teach the wrong association with sucking and feeding; they encourage comfort sucking, create wind and can make digestive issues worse, not to mention the settling problems they can create.

A newborn is not born wanting to suck to sleep and does not naturally suck for comfort – this only happens at about three months when teething starts and your baby begins to have more control over his hands and is able to put a hand to his mouth and use it as a chew toy. If your baby is comforted by a dummy during the newborn stage, it's likely that the dummy is masking an issue, as well as teaching your baby the wrong sucking associations. A well-fed baby who is wind-free and not fed on breast milk loaded with French onion soup will not want to suck after a feed or suck for comfort! Your baby will not want or need to suck to sleep if allowed awake time to digest his milk and his stomach is therefore comfortable before a nap. Your baby should not need a dummy or be rocked to settle to sleep if all the above needs are met.

Dummies create wind which interferes with a baby's immature digestive system. Sucking may pacify your baby temporarily but long-term it causes issues around settling and sleep, digestion, feeding and behaviour. A newborn will show signs of hunger if he is hungry, windy or tired – confusing, eh?! When trying to work out your baby's needs, it's always a process of elimination so make sure you are on top of your baby's milk intake, have winded him thoroughly and have allowed him enough awake time during the day.

Instead of giving your baby a dummy after a feed, make sure you have filled your baby and satisfied his hunger.

Instead of giving your baby a dummy between feeds, make sure you have winded him well and have not eaten anything that would interfere with his digestion. Giving a dummy between feeds encourages comfort sucking and exhausts the sucking action so your baby will be less inclined to actively feed and will not have the enthusiasm for feeding.

Instead of giving your baby a dummy at night to prolong sleep, increase the quantity of milk he takes during his day feeds and increase his awake time. Teach your baby self-settling techniques (see page 18) as using a dummy to settle him will not only interfere with feeds but it could mean that you are constantly up during the night putting the dummy back in your baby's mouth when it falls out. Dummy use can also interfere with your baby's appetite during the day resulting in frequent waking at night.

Using a dummy with babies who have digestive issues such as reflux can make the symptoms much worse as sucking stimulates gastric juices which stimulate acid production, causing tummy pain. Spacing out your baby's feeds – as outlined on my routine – to allow his stomach to empty between feeds, not allowing your baby to 'snack' while feeding and not using a dummy is best for your baby's digestive comfort.

Always use my three-point checklist to determine if your baby's needs have been met:

1. He is fed until full.
2. He has been winded regularly during and after feeds.
3. He has been allowed structured awake time in order to digest his milk before a nap and has had awake time during daylight hours.

A baby is always happy and sleeps well if these three needs are met.

In short ...

- Effective winding is vital for a happy baby and a good night's sleep for all.
- Trapped wind, not alleviated during feeds, can be very uncomfortable. The air in the stomach passes through the

intestines, causing pain, and passes through the other end by the next feed.

- Trapped wind forms a big air bubble in your baby's stomach, which can come up explosively bringing milk with it, resulting in projectile vomiting. If this happens, make sure you wind your baby more frequently.
- Make sure your baby's back is straight and he is wide awake when you wind him.
- Pat and rub your baby's back firmly in a circular motion, with your supporting hand putting pressure on his stomach. Be careful that you don't stroke your baby to sleep instead of winding him.
- If your baby is very windy/uncomfortable look for other reasons for discomfort, such as fast-flowing milk, comfort sucking or your own diet.
- 'Snacking', topping up between feeds as a way to settle, and therefore giving extra snacks between feeds, or using a dummy can create digestive issues and interfere with your baby's feeding routine. Allow space between feeds for your baby's stomach to fully digest and build an appetite for a meal not a snack.
- A baby crying towards the end of the day is often a symptom of wind build-up or, if you are breastfeeding, hunger. Your milk supply depletes throughout the day so follow my tips on increasing your milk supply (page 29) and supplement with a bottle of expressed milk or formula by topping up at feed times.
- If your baby is still crying excessively during and after feeds, consider other possible causes, such as reflux, lactose intolerance or cow's milk protein allergy.

PART ONE

Breastfeeding

Chapter Two

Breastfeeding: the Facts

Nowadays there seems to be so much pressure on mums to breastfeed, but very little practical advice is given. In my late mother's day, you were introduced to your midwife in early pregnancy and she advised you before, during and after the birth of your baby, giving consistent care and advice. You would spend a week in hospital being taught breastfeeding skills and baby care. By the time I started working with babies, you still saw a midwife before, during and after birth, but it was not always the same one, and you would spend three days in hospital. Fast forward 20 years and you will be lucky to see the same midwife twice, you are kicked out of hospital within 24 hours and told to feed on demand or whenever your baby 'shows signs of hunger'. Interestingly, this is not the advice given for multiple births, when you are told the opposite and to routine feed.

It is clear to me that the reduction of care given post-pregnancy is due to a lack of funding and staffing in hospitals, and mothers are no longer taught about their breasts, lactation and how to feed their babies properly. In an attempt to encourage women to breastfeed without giving practical advice, the blanket advice to feed 'on demand' is given. In my opinion this leads to so many women giving up on breast-feeding very early on or looking for some kind of structure in the first months of parenthood. The feed on demand advice would possibly work better if women were taught about lactation and how their breasts work. If you feed properly by draining both breasts at each feed, and not just offering 'snacks', then your baby would demand milk every 3–4 hours and less frequently at night, not every two hours day and night, which is so common and can leave a mother exhausted and producing less milk as a result of having so little sleep. Women stop breastfeeding for a variety of reasons, such as not knowing how much milk their baby is getting, sore and painful nipples, and exhaustion from feeding for hours at a time or feeding too frequently day and night for weeks.

It is important to go into breastfeeding with an open mind. Ninety-nine per cent of mothers I help successfully breastfeed, but it's really not the end of the world if you have to top up with a bottle. Of course breast milk is best for your baby, having been designed that way, but mixed feeding is better than no breast milk at all, and if you really can't breastfeed, remember that hundreds of babies have been brought up on formula milk alone and are fit and healthy. Above all, you have to do what is right for you; a happy mum equals a happy baby. But do give yourself a chance before deciding to stop breastfeeding – it can take a while to get established. As well as having to wait for your milk to 'come in' after the birth, which can take up to 10 days though most often it is 48 hours, you and your baby need time to get used to the whole process.

Milk Supply

Breastfeeding is a beautiful, bonding experience. In reality however, it is not so glamorous to start with and doesn't always come naturally – your breasts work in a way which is personal to you and your milk supply may change with every baby you have. Some women are blessed with the milk supply of a dairy cow while others struggle for weeks to meet their baby's demand. Your milk supply will go up and down depending on how tired you are and how much energy you are using. Some babies are naturals at latching on and drinking, while others barely open their mouths and fall asleep at the mere sniff of Mum's breast. The flow of milk is not only personal to you but can also differ between breasts. Both you and your baby have to learn breastfeeding skills together. It is often a guessing game of how much milk your baby is drinking, so getting to know your breasts and what you are supplying is essential. It can take weeks getting established with supply and demand, and often a baby's demand is way ahead of Mum's supply.

Your body first uses energy to recover from giving birth, second for daily activity and last for lactation, so establishing and maintaining a good milk supply will make all the difference to the success of feeding and your baby's routine. The Sleeping Baby Routine helps you to get one step ahead, so when the three-, six- and twelve-week growth spurts hit, you have enough milk to accommodate your baby's changing needs.

Here are several things you can do to help increase your milk supply:

- Rest during the day
- Go to bed early to get 7–8 hours' sleep, even taking into account getting up for night feeds
- Have skin-on-skin contact with your baby
- Express milk
- Drink fennel tea
- Drink 2–3 litres of water every day
- Eat well and between each breastfeed
- Actively feed and drain each breast at each feed

Rest and skin-on-skin contact

The most important thing you can do to increase your milk supply is rest. It is no coincidence that your milk supply is at its best in the morning, after a good night's sleep. Having longer stretches of sleep at night is as much of a benefit, if not more beneficial, to your supply than your breasts being stimulated at night with lots of feeding. Your milk supply naturally depletes throughout the day so having at least one good nap during the day can really give your breasts a boost. Having a skin-on-skin cuddle/nap with your baby will increase it even further with milk-making hormones being released while your baby sleeps naked (nappy on!) on your chest. General daily activities can burn up your milk supply, especially if you are running around after older children. Try having at least one 1½–2-hour rest during the day, even if you don't feel like it; take some light reading somewhere quiet and see if you drift off. Make sure you go to bed early – don't be tempted to wait up for your baby's first night feed. Your body is being worked more than it's used to; healing and recovering from birth takes energy away from lactation and you will be getting less sleep than usual due to night waking. Your body needs extra sleep during the day to compensate.

Skin-on-skin naps

I encourage a skin-on-skin nap once a day or at least once every two days. Prop yourself in an elevated position with pillows under your arms, so you are unable to roll, and tuck yourself into bed with your baby naked (leave her nappy on!) lying on your chest and enjoy a snooze together. Get everything you need around you as you won't be able to move for the duration of the nap. Babies find it hard to wake from skin-on-skin naps so wake her up five minutes earlier, allowing 15–20 minutes to wake before feeding. (See page 197 for more on skin-on-skin naps.)

Expressing

The general advice given by midwives and health visitors within the NHS is to not express in the first 4–6 weeks as it will interfere with your natural milk supply. This is fine if you are feeding on demand every few hours, day and night, but my routine is about encouraging a good milk supply so that your baby has the majority of her milk in daylight hours. In my experience, the majority of breastfeeding mothers will need a little helping hand to get one step ahead of their baby's milk demand. With supply and demand, the demand comes first (stimulation) and the supply a few days later, so the aim is to achieve a milk supply that meets and, if possible, is ahead of your baby's demand.

As your milk supply depletes naturally during the day, the Sleeping Baby Routine introduces a bottle of expressed breast milk, collected throughout the day, at the last feed of the day. This bedtime bottle is key to the success of my routine. You could use formula milk for this feed if you wish as it can take some weeks for your breasts to produce enough expressed milk for the bedtime bottle-feed. Even so, expressing your breast milk after the morning feeds will help to increase your milk supply. By expressing directly after a feed you are tricking your breasts into thinking your baby is demanding more milk. The best time to do this is after the first two morning feeds, straight after or up to 20 minutes from the end of the feed. Don't be downhearted if you get a mere 15ml (½oz) at first; it will improve and you will be stimulating your breasts regardless. By expressing straight after a feed you are also not taking the milk your breasts are producing for your baby's next feed, but instead are draining the breasts and extracting any hindmilk left, which will eventually make for more fast-flowing milk. Do not express before a feed.

The best way to express is to do a few minutes each side several times. When the milk flow stops, change to the other side. For efficient expressing use a double pump and start the full cycle 2–3 times on as high a setting as is comfortable. This will be more stimulating than leaving the pump running for 10–20 minutes. Hold the pump funnels in the natural position of your breasts, aligning them with whatever direction your nipples face (be that straight ahead, east, west or downwards!), and focus on what is happening. For the last five minutes, swap to a single pump, massage different areas of your breast and observe which areas release milk. (Once you have found your 'hotspots' for releasing more milk, you can use this massaging technique for the last five minutes of feeding your baby to encourage sucking and to help drain and extract the stubborn hindmilk.) Massage from the armpit and under the breast and squeeze gently to encourage drainage. The hindmilk is the thick, creamy milk which is slower in flow and sometimes hard for a baby to extract. Breast milk flow is personal to you and some breasts will release milk all in one hit and then stop, while others will release milk in spurts. Keep the pump going slightly longer (2–3 minutes) than the flow of milk to make sure you are completely drained. I recommend either the Lansinoh 2 in 1 double electric breast pump, which has a battery pack and is portable with a handy timer, or the Medela Freestyle, or you can hire the Medela Symphony Double which is the mother of all pumps! (Search online for your nearest available agent.)

Water and fennel tea

Drink plenty of water: you should have 2–3 litres per day. Try to remember to put a jug of water and a glass next to your chair before feeding, so that you can sip water as you go along. Sipping water gradually, instead of knocking back pints in one go, means the water will hold in your system instead of it flushing through and making you want to go to the loo every five minutes. Eating plenty of fruit and vegetables will mean your body will retain more water.

Drinking herbal tea also counts as your water intake, and drinking fennel tea in particular helps to increase your milk supply – have a cup at each feed using two bags for extra strength, along with your water. Fennel tea has the added benefit of helping to soothe your baby's digestive tract (via your milk). There are also a few other breastfeeding teas out there that may help, but I've always found that fennel tea works best.

Eating for breastfeeding

It is so important that you eat regularly and give yourself enough time between feeds to digest this food before your baby's next feed. You need about 300–500 extra calories a day when breast-feeding. Your baby is eating what you are eating so making your diet nutritionally dense and increasing the quality of your food intake will satisfy her. I looked after one mum many moons ago who had plenty of milk, but she couldn't understand why her baby wasn't sleeping well, day or night. It turned out that she was skipping meals and eating a tiny amount when she did eat – fewer than 1,000 calories a day – to get her pre-baby body back as quickly as possible! If she had eaten more, her milk would have satisfied her baby for longer and he would have slept longer at night and more peacefully during the day. You really do need to eat three meals a day, have healthy snacks between meals and, again, drink, drink, drink!

Dieting while breastfeeding is a no-no I'm afraid! Your baby will get out what you put in – feed your milk to feed your baby – so if you are not eating regularly and living on lettuce leaves, this will not fill your baby up and can affect your milk production. I'm not saying that you need to eat the whole biscuit barrel either, but a healthy balance and choosing the right foods will help you feel and stay healthy, increase your milk supply and improve the quality of your milk. Even if you have a lot of milk, it doesn't always mean it is good-quality milk. Eating the right foods also has a positive effect on your mood and can help stabilise your blood sugar, which will be very useful if you are tired and sleep-deprived. Breastfeeding can help you lose your baby weight, but most mothers will naturally hold on to some weight until they stop breastfeeding.

Your baby is eating what you eat and is born with an immature gut that is usually sensitive and will react to wind-forming foods. Eating these foods can cause havoc with digestion and disrupt your baby's sleep patterns and the quantity of milk she takes. The foods below should be avoided in the first six weeks of your baby's life while you are establishing the routine. If your baby is very sensitive and you are having a hard time winding her, check food labels for hidden ingredients; most ready meals and soups contain onion.

Foods to avoid for the first six weeks:

- Spices
- Chilli
- Peppers
- Onion family: onions, leeks, spring onions
- Cabbage family, cauliflower and broccoli
- Lettuce: particularly those with lighter green leaves. Spinach, for example, rarely causes problems
- Cucumber
- Rocket
- Beans, lentils and pulses
- Acidic foods, such as tomatoes, berries and oranges: too much acidity in your diet can cause diarrhoea and a sore bottom for your baby
- Caffeine: coffee, tea and other caffeinated food and drinks can affect your baby's sleep pattern. Try to limit caffeine to the mornings and replace your tea or coffee with a cup of fennel tea
- Alcohol is, of course, off-limits

If you think that a particular food has upset your baby, remember that it takes 4–6 hours after you eat for a food to affect your breast milk. Try eliminating the food you suspect from your diet for a minimum of 1–2 weeks before trying it again.

If you think that your baby is reacting to dairy, feeds are becoming problematic or your baby is refusing the breast and vomiting, then try cutting out all dairy but be sure to eat other foods that are high in calcium, such as broccoli, nuts, spinach and tinned salmon. Swap cow's milk for almond, coconut or rice milk and eat goat's cheese instead of cow's milk cheese.

Avocados and nuts are a good source of healthy fats. Don't shy away from healthy fat as it won't make you fat! It's the sugar that's evil and has little nutritional value.

Excessive fruits, such as tomatoes, berries and soft fruits, can make babies' bottoms sore, though this is not the case for all babies. If you notice a red bottom, stick to pears, apples and bananas.

I'm all about healthy and nutritionally-dense eating even with my own diet. I don't like processed foods but I understand that it can be hard to make time to prepare nutritional, balanced meals for yourself when you are trying to get to grips with parenthood. Try these quick snack ideas if you are short on time or inspiration:

- A bowl of mixed nuts
- Scrambled or poached eggs, or an omelette: eggs are a good source of protein
- Rice/corn cakes or Ryvita with cottage cheese and tomato, or peanut butter
- Wholemeal pitta bread stuffed with ham, salmon or tuna with salad; oily fish, such as salmon and mackerel, are a good source of vitamins A and D, as well as omega-3, which is good for the quality of your milk and your baby's development. Limit your intake of oily fish to two portions a week as it can contain low levels of pollutants
- Avocado and smoked salmon on sourdough toast with olive oil, black pepper and lime
- Steak and spinach will give you an iron boost

- Jacket potato or baked sweet potato with healthy fillings, such as prawns and avocado, cottage cheese and grated carrot, or feta cheese, tomato and olives

You could also try making a salad bowl with rice or pasta at the beginning of the day to dip into throughout the day. Make sure you leave out the wind-forming foods mentioned on page 34. I like to make a big bowl of salad using spinach, tomato, cucumber, beetroot, carrot, pumpkin seeds and avocado with a wedge of lime – yummy!

While you are breastfeeding it is so important to ensure you are getting enough calcium and iron by eating lots of spinach and broccoli. I love my blender and I cram it full of goodies for a breastfeeding smoothie: almond or coconut milk, banana, berries, nuts and seeds.

A good balanced diet will make great quality milk without meaning that you put on weight, but if you fancy the odd cream doughnut – why not? You deserve it!

Active feeding

By teaching your baby to associate your breast with food and feeding, not with comfort sucking and/or as an aid to sleep, will ultimately increase your supply because your breasts will be properly stimulated and drained. Active sucking makes for efficient feeding and a well-fed baby. Conversely, comfort sucking and snoozing leads to less milk intake and resultant disrupted sleep due to hunger and catnapping on the breast. Comfort sucking looks like a short up-and-down action, often with a shuddery jaw – nibble, nibble, pause, or long pause with the occasional suck. Active feeding looks like a wide circular motion with visible swallowing. Babies will naturally slow down as the milk flow slows, so encourage your baby to drain the breast and not slow down until her time is up or your breast is empty. Do this by tickling her feet, neck and tummy. It is hard for a newborn to stay awake while feeding.

The sucking action alone is tiring in the first weeks of life and it's common for newborns to close their eyes while feeding. If they are still actively sucking, that is fine, but as they slow down or comfort suck they will drift off to sleep. The comfort of being in a cuddle-like position makes it difficult for a baby to resist a catnap, so it's important to prompt your baby to keep her actively sucking for the duration of the feed. A build-up of wind can also cause comfort sucking, which is why it is so important to regularly wind your baby (see page 7).

Active feeding also encourages your baby to only associate sucking with feeding and not with sleep, which will help with self-settling in the long-term.

Milk Intake and Quantities

Milk intake with breastfeeding is always a guesstimate. However, the general advice for a baby's daily milk intake is around 200ml (7oz) of milk per kilogram of body weight. So if your newborn is 4kg (8lb 13oz), in 24 hours she will need 800ml (28oz) of milk. This is a rough guide and some babies who are growing at a fast rate or have a bigger appetite will take more milk at each feed.

The amount of milk your baby drinks in 24 hours is personal to her and will increase gradually until her intake plateaus once she is sleeping through the night and her growth slows. Whether you divide your baby's milk intake into six or 10 feeds, the total daily amount will still be the same. The idea is to give your baby larger feeds during the day and increase these feeds gradually while capping the quantity at the night feeds, and then decreasing the quantity at the night feeds as she gradually sleeps later through the night. With the decrease of milk intake during the night, the day feeds eventually take on the entire milk needed in a 24-hour period.

This is not about getting as much milk as possible into your baby at each feed in order to encourage her to sleep through the night. Rather it is about making sure she is full at each feed and gradually increasing the quantity of milk she is regularly taking until she is sleeping through the night. This regular intake at each feed should always increase and not decrease during the day but your baby will not be able to take any increase larger than 15–30ml (½–1oz) at a time. It's worth noting that some babies of a smaller weight can have a larger appetite than a bigger baby. I'm a twin specialist and quite often look after twins where the smaller twin, weighing a whole 0.45kg (1lb) less than the other twin, drinks more milk in 24 hours than her larger sibling, having a bigger appetite while catching up and growing fast.

Overfeeding on a routine is unlikely as feeds are structured; it's when parents feed their baby on demand and offer milk for comfort – to settle and soothe – as well as for hunger, regardless of the guidelines for milk intake, that overfeeding becomes an issue. You should follow your baby's appetite and what she needs as an individual. By 4–8 weeks, babies in my care are sleeping through the night. These babies will be taking 730–1040ml (25–36oz) of milk per 24 hours and generally weigh around 3.17–4.9kg (7–11lb).

Breast Health

Nipples

Breastfeeding isn't supposed to hurt, but most mothers will get some nipple soreness during the early stages of nursing. It's not unusual to feel some discomfort when your baby first latches on, especially in the first few weeks. Latching can cause a pain that mothers have described as pins going through their nipples. The sensation should die off after a minute or so as your baby sucks. The time it takes for the pain to reduce lessens and soon disappears altogether by Weeks 2–3.

Your nipples are a very sensitive part of your body and are not used to being munched. It's not surprising, then, that it takes a while for your delicate nipple tissue to adapt. Sore, painful nipples can make breastfeeding torture and, if the soreness continues, there may be some other cause for it, such as:

- incorrect positioning and poor latch
- prolonged feeding and comfort sucking
- cracks and infection, such as thrush or mastitis (see below)

Protecting your nipples is essential for at least the first month. Creams to protect and keep your nipples moist, such as Lansinoh Nipple Cream, are great for keeping your nipples supple. If you have damaged nipples with soreness or cracks, one of the best treatments is Jelonet gauze, which is usually used for burns but is fantastic at healing nipples. Cut the gauze into squares and place them in the fridge. Use at bedtime or when you have a long gap between feeds and wash off before feeding.

Breast lumps

Lumpy breasts, red patches and blocked ducts are common when breastfeeding. Check your breasts every day so you get to know how they feel when breastfeeding. Most breasts feel lumpy, especially around the armpit glands. Lumps are common especially when your breasts are full. These lumps are caused by blocked milk ducts. Lumps can also appear if your bra does not fit well and presses into your breast. Massaging your breast towards the end of each breastfeed will help release any stubborn milk, help drain your ducts and help your newborn reach the hindmilk (see page 32 for advice on how to do this). Hard or small lumps are common, but if they are particularly stubborn or are causing soreness, use a warm compress while feeding. Lumps and breast tissue changes are normal and are not always a sign of infection, and if massaged out shouldn't cause any problems. If your baby hasn't drained the lumpy side, then express it out. A massage in a warm shower or bath will help, as will a hot flannel compress while feeding.

Mastitis

Mastitis is an inflammation of the breast. Mastitis can also be caused by exhaustion, blocked ducts or by an infection passed through the nipple which travels into the milk ducts. Bacteria are not always present, and antibiotics may not be needed if self-help measures are started straight away. Massage your breasts, rest between feeds and ensure your baby drains your breasts (see page 45). Doing this can prevent an infection occurring. If you start to feel flu-like symptoms, such as aches and pains, a fever, shivering, being tearful, hot breasts or feeling exhausted, you have developed an infection. At the first sign of this, go straight to bed and take paracetamol every four hours (but no more than four doses in 24 hours) to try and combat the symptoms. If the symptoms do not subside within 24 hours you will need to see your GP who will prescribe antibiotics. Do not stop breastfeeding during this time as draining your breasts and therefore unblocking the ducts will help with recovery. Start feeding on the breast that has mastitis to make sure it is drained thoroughly. The infection will not be passed to your baby.

If you have to take antibiotics, take a high-strength probiotic after your course has finished. Antibiotics kill natural bacteria in the body, lower your immune system, reduce your milk supply and can give your baby a stomach ache.

Position and Latching

Poor positioning of your baby's mouth over the nipple can cause prolonged pain and soreness while feeding. First, you need to be in the correct position yourself. Make sure you are sitting up straight and perhaps use a footstool if your feet are not flat on the floor. Get in a position where you are comfortable without holding any tension which can stop your milk flow. Before you start feeding, take a deep breath, squeeze your shoulders up towards your ears, then breathe out and relax your shoulders down, though I appreciate this can sometimes be tricky when you have a baby screaming at you wanting milk!

Try not to hunch over – I know this is a temptation as you look down lovingly at your new baby and to push your nipple into her mouth, but you need to bring your baby's head and mouth towards your nipple, not the other way around. Sit with your back straight, not leaning back. A breastfeeding

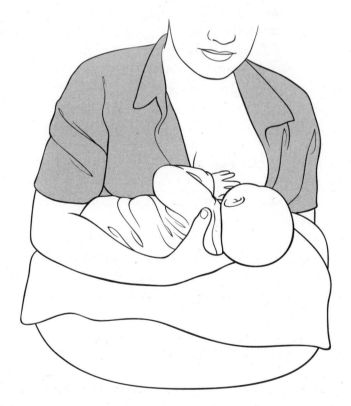

Breastfeeding with nursing pillow

cushion will help you get the right height. I love the 'My Brest Friend' or 'Doomoo' nursing pillows which support your back and leave your hands free to tickle your baby and encourage feeding. Your baby needs to have a nice wide open mouth to latch properly and as far over the areola (the dark area around the nipple) as possible, pointing your nipple into the roof of her mouth. To encourage her to do this, tease the nipple across her top lip, under her nose, so her top lip has to come up and over the nipple. If your nipples face slightly 'east' or 'west', or if you are feeding twins, the rugby/football position may be best for you.

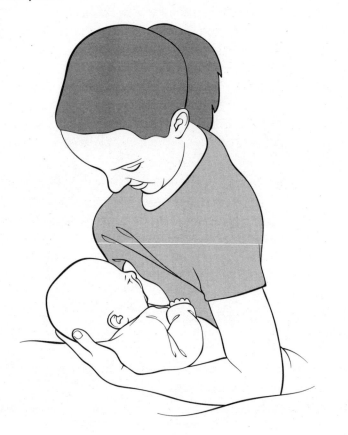

Breastfeeding in football/rugby hold

Inverted nipples

When your breasts become engorged and ready to breastfeed, your nipples tend to protrude. Inverted nipples, however, can take much longer to be coaxed out. Breastfeeding with inverted nipples is not impossible, but you will need to work at it.

Nipple shields are often recommended to help draw out the nipple. Usually this is all they do, as it is very hard for a baby to draw milk through a shield and to stimulate the nipple. Allow your baby to suck at the shield for 30–60 seconds to draw your nipple out then quickly remove it and latch your baby on to the nipple while it's still drawn out.

Expressing for 30–60 seconds before a feed to draw out the nipple is probably easier and more effective than using nipple shields, but you will have to latch your baby on very quickly while the nipple is drawn out. Hold your breast and make a protruding teat-like shape with your nipple so your baby can latch. If possible, hold the shape by squeezing just over the nipple for a couple of minutes while your baby is sucking. The use of ice cubes to harden the nipple can also help. This technique also works for babies with tongue tie, a high palate or recessed jaw, all of which make hard work of latching.

Problems latching your baby on to inverted nipples should ease with time as your nipples get used to being used and regularly drawn out. Experiment with different positions, such as the rugby/football position on page 42.

So there you have the facts about breastfeeding ... Now let's get your breasts working and help you establish breastfeeding! From the first latch to actually having a milk supply can take some weeks. Follow my simple plan in the next chapter for maximum breast stimulation balanced with enough rest to recover from birth and care for your nipples.

Chapter Three

Establishing Breastfeeding

The advice in this chapter is designed to allow you to establish a good milk supply before moving on to my standard 7pm to 7am Sleeping Baby Routine (Chapters Four and Five), which will see you through until the weaning stage (at 4–6 months).

There is so much conflicting advice out there on breastfeeding. Firstly, when breastfeeding you should be offering your baby both breasts at each feed. This is not only to stimulate, increase and maintain your milk supply, but also to ensure that your baby is full after each feed. You should also alternate the breast you start with at each feed. This ensures that each breast is emptied at least every other feed. Your baby (or you!) may tend to favour one breast which can often produce more milk than the other or is easier to latch on to. If you always start on the favoured breast you could end up with one breast larger than the other and produce much more milk on the favoured side, so make sure you swap the starter breast at each feed.

The First 24–48 Hours: Stimulation and Establishing Lactation

Before your breasts start to produce milk, you will produce colostrum, a thick yellowish or clear sticky liquid. This is top-quality, powerful stuff – high in protein and packed full of antibodies. It also has a laxative effect to help push out your baby's meconium stools. It is important to regularly stimulate your breasts with short, active bursts of feeding while in the first few days of producing colostrum.

In order to stimulate your milk production, offer your baby short bursts of 10–15 minutes of active feeding on each breast every 1–2 hours during the day for the first 24–48 hours. This is to give frequent active stimulation during the day which encourages lactation. After 9/10pm let your baby sleep for longer if he wants to as this will also give you the rest needed after giving birth, which is as much a benefit to your milk supply as frequent sucking. Encouraging longer gaps between feeds at night and a greater intake of milk and feeds during the day will also help your baby to quickly establish the difference between night and day. If you are uncomfortable with leaving your newborn to wake naturally for a feed, you can feed him every 4–5 hours during the night until the morning. However, it is unlikely that your baby will sleep for any length of time at night at this stage and will wake when he is hungry.

Feeding your baby every 1–2 hours during the day and 4+ hourly at night will be more stimulating for your breasts than leaving him to suck or comfort suck on an empty breast. Common advice is to let your newborn feed as long as he wants to, whenever he wants to. In my experience, the trouble with this is, if there is no milk to drink, sucking for long periods on an empty breast can make your nipples very sore and damaged by the time your milk actually does come in. This is also not 'active stimulation' so won't have the same impact as active sucking frequently for shorter bursts, as my routine encourages.

It can take from 24 hours to 10 days for your milk to 'come in', so how long you stay on this routine will depend on when this happens. Signs that your milk has come in are:

- you become temporarily engorged
- your breasts swell and become hard
- your milk turns a milky-white colour

Once your milk has come in

When your milk has come in, extend the time on each breast to 20–30 minutes at each feed, feeding three-hourly during the day. If your baby is over 2.72kg (6lb), is feeding well during the day and is going over four hours between feeds at night, letting him naturally wake is fine as long as he is gaining weight. Leaving longer periods between feeds at night will mean that you get more rest, which is essential for recovery and producing milk. Some women start lactating within 24 hours but it can take up to 10 days for your milk to come in, especially if you've had a C-section.

Some babies are born sleepy and not so hungry, while others are ravenous. If the latter, giving a little formula of 30ml (1oz) maximum in the first 48 hours will not only satisfy your baby overnight but will give you much-needed sleep to recover and help encourage your milk supply. This will also save your nipples from being damaged due to lengthy sucking on empty breasts. In my experience, giving formula through a bottle will not discourage a baby from the breast if given in very small, controlled quantities, but instead will give the breasts a chance to rest and do what they need to do to start producing milk. Formula is best given in the evening so as to not interfere with your daily stimulation and to allow you both to get some sleep. Of course, if you give your baby too much formula, he will be disinterested in latching on to the breast when you want him to. Like everything, it's all about balance.

Check your breasts for milk to gauge if you have any milk left (see box below) whenever you break to wind your baby, which should be after every 5–10 minutes of active sucking, or if your baby has fallen asleep or is comfort sucking. If your baby is sleepy and inactive during a day feed, make sure you express to keep stimulation up and encourage your milk supply (see page 30 for more on this).

How to check your breasts for milk

Squeeze through the breast to the nipple with your forefinger and thumb. If milk is released easily your breast may not be empty and you should offer your baby five more minutes on that side, and then check again. You should spend a maximum of 30 minutes on each breast. Some mothers will always have a little milk left whenever they check as they are constantly producing, but for most this is a great way of checking if your breasts are empty. Test this method by expressing straight after feeding to see how much milk you have left. If it is less than 30ml (1oz) then your baby has drained your breast.

Active feeding

The objective is to teach your baby that your breasts are for feeding and not for comfort or for inducing sleep, which can be tricky in the first six weeks of life as your baby snuggles into your body and the soporific action of sucking alone makes it very hard for him to stay awake. I often see parents trying to wake their baby by patting, rocking or jiggling them around, which will have the opposite effect and will send a baby to sleep. Background noise, such as the radio, TV, chatting or kitchen appliances, will also lull a baby to sleep. Newborns are heat-, light- and sound-sensitive (see page 188).

Below are some tips on encouraging active and wakeful feeding:

- Wake your baby 10–15 minutes before each day feed and strip him down to just his vest bodysuit in order to cool his body temperature down in preparation for the feed. Tickling his hands and feet will help with waking.

48

- Keep your baby cool while feeding. At a room temperature of 19–20°C a vest bodysuit is all the clothing needed. A baby's body will heat up while breastfeeding and digesting and being close to Mum. Don't worry if your baby's feet and hands feel or look cool, it's the warmth of his body you need to check.
- A cool water nappy change usually helps wake a snoozy baby.
- Tickle your baby's hands and feet, and anywhere you find sensitive, to help keep him actively feeding and to help with waking for winding.
- A newborn often won't be able to stay sucking actively while breastfeeding for longer than 5–10 minutes at a time. Place your baby down on a muslin square or towel on the floor and he will awaken more easily as he is not having bodily contact with you. Briefly laying your baby on his back also helps bring up wind (see page 12).

Winding

Always ensure you wind your baby effectively as trapped air can swell up in his tummy, making him feel unnaturally full and sleepy (see page 7 for more on this). Wind your baby every 5–10 minutes or when feeding has naturally slowed down. Always wake your baby before winding as it is virtually impossible to wind a sleeping baby. Newborns often grunt and make throaty noises which can be mistaken for burps – you should be able to hear a burp clearly when you have successfully released the trapped wind. Bear in mind that some babies will let out a single large and guttural burp, while others will release two or three smaller burps. In time you will get to know what is normal for your baby.

> ## Keep a baby routine diary
>
> Keeping a baby diary will help you to remember which breast you last fed on (especially when it is 3am and you can't remember!) and will allow you to log your baby's feeds (the start time and duration), any winding details, his daily awake time, your milk supply and the expressing time, length and quantity.

Week 1: Three-hourly Feeding

This routine is to be followed *during the first week of life only*, feeding three-hourly as your milk starts to come in.

Time the feeds from the start of each feed, running from 6am to 9pm, or 7am to 10pm, and then four- to five-hourly thereafter during the night. If your baby is over 2.72kg (6lb) and is gaining weight you can leave him to wake naturally. Feed your baby for 20–30 minutes on each side, which includes winding, and 15 minutes each side for night feeds. If for some reason your baby is too tired or unable to take both breasts, express the side that has not been drained so that both breasts are being stimulated and drained every three hours during the day. This will encourage a good milk supply – in the first week of lactation it is all down to stimulation and draining the milk you are producing.

Stay on this routine until you have established a milk supply, your baby is over 2.72kg (6lb) and is gaining weight. You can then follow the routines outlined in Chapter Four.

Three-hourly Feeds While Establishing Breastfeeding	
6am	Start on left breast Feed for 20–30 minutes each side Total awake time (including feed): 1–1½ hours

7/7.30am	Nap
9am	Start on right breast Feed for 20–30 minutes each side Total awake time (including feed): 1–1½ hours
10/10.30am	Nap
12pm	Start on left breast Feed for 20–30 minutes each side Total awake time (including feed): 1–1½ hours
1/1.30pm	Nap
3pm	Start on right breast Feed for 20–30 minutes each side Total awake time (including feed): 1–1½ hours
4/4.30pm	Nap
6pm	Left breast only Feed for 20–30 minutes
6.30pm	Bath (34–35°C) or strip wash and change for the night
6.45pm	Right breast only Feed for 20–30 minutes
7.15pm	Nap
9/9.15pm	Start on left breast Feed for 20 minutes each side
9.40/10pm	Bedtime (swaddled)
During the night	Feed for 15 minutes each side whenever your baby wakes (night-time feeds are kept much smaller) Change your baby's nappy before the feed

Notes on routine

- Wake your newborn 10–15 minutes before each feed to ensure he is wide awake and enthusiastic before going on to the breast. Strip off his sleepsuit/Babygro and feed in just a vest bodysuit; babies get very warm while breastfeeding.

- Alternate the breast you start on at each feed. Before changing to the second breast, check your breast for milk (see page 48). If you still have milk, give another five minutes on the first side before checking again. Change to the other breast when you have run out of milk on the first side or when your baby has been feeding for 30 minutes.
- Change your baby's nappy *after* feeds during the day – most babies dirty their nappies while feeding. If you do change before a feed, change the nappy again after the feed to ensure the nappy lasts through to the next feed. (See page 167 for more on nappy changing.)
- Change your baby's nappy *before* feeds during the night to help avoid stimulation after the feed and aid a smooth transition back to bed.
- Swaddling for the last five minutes of a night feed will also help a smooth settling process. Get your baby's wind up using the over-the-shoulder position (page 10) and then put him back to bed.
- Keep night feeds dark (barely lit) and quiet.
- Winding properly is very important, so take another look at Chapter One for help with getting this right. Make sure your baby is wide awake while winding and feeding as it's almost impossible to wind a sleeping baby. Wind your baby every 5–10 minutes while feeding if active sucking has slowed or to help wake your baby if he falls asleep.
- In the first week of life, you are unlikely to be able to keep your baby awake long enough to have any real awake time, but if he is in fact able to do so then allow no more than 1½ hours timed from the start of the feed. Feeding every three hours means he is already having a lot of activity, being woken for feeds, and will need at least 1½–2 hours' sleep between daytime feeds. He should, however, be able to stay awake for the one-hour feed period. Structured play/awake time will start when you move on to the more realistic 3½–4-hourly feeding routine (Chapter Four).

Gilly's five-day consultation

Monday

Gilly is three weeks old but was born four weeks premature and weighs 2.46kg (5lb 7oz). To help Gilly gain
weight, on leaving hospital Antonia (Gilly's mum) was
advised to not let Gilly go more than three hours between
feeds. Gilly was therefore being fed every three hours day
and night and had reached a great weight of over 3.17kg
(7lb). I have cared for hundreds of premature babies and,
if they are gaining weight and Mum's milk supply is ahead
of baby's demand, there is no reason why, if the baby is
over 2.72kg (6lb), they cannot be put straight on to
my 7pm–7am routine.

My advice to Antonia on leaving hospital would have
been to feed Gilly every three hours for a 12-hour day
and then every 4–5 hours during the night, which would
have given Antonia rest and encouraged Gilly to have
longer stretches of sleep during the night. This would
have made day feeds more effective, not to mention
teaching Gilly the difference between day and night from
the off. Gilly, having been woken every three hours
during the day and night, was understandably exhausted,
not feeding well and was falling asleep while being
breastfed. As a result she was too tired to take a full feed
during the day and then was not sleeping well day or
night because of her low milk intake and reliance on
several feeds at night to reach the milk intake needed for
her age and weight.

Exhausted and distraught, Antonia contacted me.
Firstly I advised her to stop waking Gilly at night and to
let her wake of her own accord. Having lower milk intake
at night would naturally increase her appetite, and therefore her milk intake during the day, and would also give
her enough sleep to be able to focus and stay awake

for day feeds as well as a little playtime. I also advised Antonia to keep feeding every three hours during the day, starting from 6am, introduce the staggered bedtime feed at 6pm, and express after the morning feeds to help increase her milk supply in preparation for moving on to the 7pm–7am routine, and to gather enough milk for the post-bath bottle.

Gilly's new routine looked like this:

6am	Breastfeed for 45–60 minutes
7am	Express for 15–20 minutes
7.30am	Nap
9am	Breastfeed for 45–60 minutes
10am	Express for 15–20 minutes
10.30/11am	Nap
12pm	Breastfeed for 45–60 minutes
1pm	Express for 10–15 minutes
1.30/2pm	Nap
3pm	Breastfeed for 45–60 minutes No express
4.30pm	Nap
6pm	Breastfeed for 20–30 minutes
6.30pm	Bath (34–35°C)
6.45pm	Bottle-feed: 60–120ml (2–4oz) expressed breast milk
7.30/8pm	Bedtime (swaddled)
During the night	Feed for 15 minutes each side (30 minutes maximum) whenever Gilly wakes

I also advised making sure Gilly was woken 15 minutes before a feed to ensure she was wide awake and ready to actively feed, and also to keep Gilly stimulated while feeding, which in turn would result in an increase of milk intake and breast stimulation.

Tuesday

I checked in with Antonia to see how the new plan was working out. Gilly had dropped a feed in the night, feeding twice instead of the usual three times. Antonia and I decided she should stay on the three-hourly feeding for another day before moving over to the 7pm–7am routine the following day and to gradually increase the post-bath, bedtime bottle by 30ml (1oz) at a time until night feeds were phased out completely.

Wednesday

Gilly woke twice in the night for a 30-minute feed at 1am and 4.30am, but was hard to settle after this later feed. We discussed keeping Gilly swaddled for feeds if she woke after 4am and to offer a shorter feed of 10–15 minutes. Gilly was also unsettled after the 3pm feed.

We moved Gilly on to the 7pm–7am routine, lengthening the time between feeds. With fewer feeds during the day it was important that Gilly was actively feeding and draining the breasts. If Gilly still looked hungry after the afternoon feed, Antonia was to offer 30–60ml (1–2oz) from a bottle as a top-up, straight after the breastfeed. On the new routine Antonia could start to gradually increase Gilly's awake time to up to two hours at each feed period.

Thursday

Gilly's bedtime bottle had increased to 150ml (5oz) and she woke once at 3am on Wednesday night. Great result! My advice was to now add an express between 8pm and 9pm, which would help maintain Antonia's milk supply and ensure she was comfortable overnight.

Friday

Gilly was well on her way to sleeping through the night and woke at 3am on Thursday night for a 20-minute feed. Increasing her awake time impacted on how much sleep she needed at night, but overall her increase of milk intake during the day was satisfying most of the milk needed in a 24-hour period. This daily volume will need to increase until she sleeps through and her growth slows down.

Although frequent feeding day and night is advised to stimulate a mother's milk supply and to help the baby gain weight, exhaustion often counteracts that effect for both mother and baby. An exhausted mother can find it hard to supply enough milk for full feeds to sustain her baby for any length of time, and the baby therefore only gets enough milk to snack frequently. The more rested the mother, the greater the milk supply to satisfy her baby's appetite. Now Gilly's mother is well-rested, sleeps eight hours at night and has enough expressed milk to store in the freezer – happy days!

Chapter Four

Weeks 2-3

Y ou have two options when your milk comes in at Week 2. If your baby is over 2.72kg (6lb) in weight, is gaining weight and is back to her birth weight, and your milk supply meets or is ahead of your baby's demand, you can move straight to the 7pm to 7am Sleeping Baby Routine (page 69).

However, if your baby has low weight gain, is not back to her birth weight and your milk supply is not yet meeting demand or is one step behind your baby's appetite then follow the three-hourly routine outlined on page 68. The benefit of this routine is that your breasts will have extra stimulation from active sucking and your baby will have an extra feed during the day until your milk supply increases. On the downside, this routine can be exhausting for you and your baby as there is less 'downtime' between feeds and the added factor of playtime and expressing means very little time is left for rest and looking after your basic needs. This routine is not practical in the long-term but it can be used until your milk supply has increased. Move on to the 7pm–7am routine as soon as you are able to. If you have a low milk supply or are not meeting your hungry baby's appetite, another option is to follow the mixed feeding routine (Chapter Six) or to temporarily mix feed on the 7pm–7am routine while increasing your milk supply.

With both routines you will now introduce a bottle at bedtime, express your breast milk to maintain and increase your milk supply, and structure some awake time for your baby at each day feed. Try to increase your baby's awake time from 1¼ to 1½ hours at a time during Weeks 2–3 and 1½ to 2 hours at a time by Weeks 4–6 (this includes feeding, winding and nappy changes, as well as playtime). Some 'widey-wakey' babies may be able to stay awake for 1½–2 hours at some feed periods from birth. However, do not let your newborn stay awake for more than two hours at any one feed. This is the maximum awake time for babies aged 1–6 weeks, as your little one also needs quality naps to ensure she has the energy to feed well and thrive.

Activity can be tiring and the amount of awake time your baby has may vary at each feed period. I work on establishing how much time an individual newborn is able to stay awake for and then build on that until two hours of awake time at each feed period is their natural pace. The idea is to encourage moving forward with the routine without backtracking. If, for several weeks, your baby is able to stay awake for two hours happily for each feed period, and then randomly starts falling asleep after an hour, you should try to encourage your baby to wake up and keep to the routine. Any extra time needed for sleep should be taken at night. If you have a sleepy baby from the start who is only able to stay awake for, say, one hour, you should build on that time and gradually encourage a longer time playing, eventually reaching two hours by Weeks 4–6.

As your baby grows she will hit growth spurts and will be wide awake and hungry for 2–4 days and then become very sleepy for a few days after, while growing. I call this a 'mini weekly growth spurt'. Your baby will have major growth spurts at around three weeks, six weeks and three months.

The bedtime bottle

Babies on my routine rarely have a problem with settling to bed at night. In fact, sometimes it's a job to keep them awake long enough after the bath to take their bottle before bed! Naturally babies become tired at this time of day and recognise that bedtime is coming. It's important that you invest time in the bedtime bottle as this will be the key to your baby sleeping through the night. It can take weeks for your newborn to become efficient at this feed, but keep with it as it will eventually all click into place. As with the other day feeds, the aim is to keep your baby actively feeding, winding and waking her if she falls asleep. At this point it's more about keeping your baby stimulated and awake to take enough milk before bed, rather than making the room dark and peaceful to help send her to sleep as you would a much older baby who is already established.

The bedtime bottle-feed, after the bath, could increase by 30–60ml (1–2oz) per week in the first month, thus becoming the biggest feed of the day, which will enable your baby to sleep for long periods at night. When you first introduce the bottle, you will not know how much milk your baby will want or need so, as a starting point, introduce the bedtime bottle with 60ml (2oz) of milk for a 2–3-week-old baby. If this is easily taken, the next night increase it to 90ml (3oz), and then gradually increase the amount until your baby reaches a comfortable intake that meets her personal appetite. Increasing by only 30ml (1oz) at a time until you have met your baby's appetite means you won't overfeed her. From there look to increase the amount gradually by 15–30ml (½–1oz) at a time until your baby has reached the amount she personally needs to sleep through the night. The quantity in the bottle really does need to increase gradually – your baby has a very small stomach. Some babies will increase slowly by 15–30ml (½–1oz) per week, while others will increase their milk intake by 60ml (2oz). This increase will slow and stop once your baby is sleeping through the night.

It's worth bearing in mind that the amount of milk needed is not always based on the weight of a baby, but also on her appetite and how quickly she is growing. I have often looked after newborn twins where the smaller twin, sometimes a whole 0.45kg (1lb) lighter than her sibling, will drink 30ml (1oz) or so more at each feed than the bigger twin, which can only be explained by a faster rate of growth and a bigger appetite.

With the bedtime bottle you will also need to be aware, and take into consideration, how much milk your baby is taking before the bath, as this will have an impact on the bedtime bottle-feed. If you are unable to increase your baby's milk intake with this bottle, then look to reduce the pre-bath breastfeed by five minutes on each breast. If you have fast-flowing milk, your baby could be getting 90–120ml (3–4oz) in as little as 10 minutes. Ideally she would be taking no more than 60ml (2oz) at the pre-bath feed.

The bedtime bottle-feed is the key to your baby sleeping through the night. Make sure you find the right teat and bottle for your baby's sucking style (see page 102) and wind her every 15–30ml (½–1oz), or even more regularly if you have a particularly windy baby. Warm the milk before giving your baby a bottle as newborns do not like drinking cold milk – it's harder to digest and can give your baby stomach ache. To test the temperature of the milk, shake some on the inside of your wrist. If it stings it is too hot; it should feel warm or you should feel nothing. You can also reheat the milk if it has cooled during the feed. Use a bottle warmer or a jug of hot water, and always test the temperature after reheating. It's commonly thought that it's a good idea not to heat a baby's milk as it risks creating a fussy feeder. However, during the newborn stage it's all about digestion, and warm milk is easier to digest. Once you reach the baby stage – from 12 weeks – your baby's gut is less sensitive and can handle cooler milk.

Maintaining your milk supply

Once your milk has come in, you will still need to maintain a good supply. To help this you need to rest, eat and drink well, and express, collecting milk for the bedtime bottle. Express for 15–20 minutes no later than 20 minutes after the two morning feeds (10 minutes if using a double pump). Any later than this and you will be expressing milk produced for the next feed and therefore depriving your baby of that milk. Have the breast pump set up and ready to go before starting feeds. Preparation will not only save you time but keep the feed and expressing within the time allocated. Add an extra express between 8pm and 9pm once your baby is waking up at night past 1am or 2am and is likely to be waking only once in the night to feed. Expressing before you go to bed will help to maintain a good milk supply and keep your breasts comfortable for you to sleep as your baby gradually wakes later through the night. Don't be tempted to add this to your routine before she is regularly waking past 1–2am otherwise you will not have enough milk for the first night feed.

A mother has her most plentiful milk supply in the morning as, in theory, she has had a good night's sleep (more sleep = more milk). During the day, milk production reduces and your supply depletes, which leaves you at the lowest point of milk supply come the evening feed. However, this is when your baby needs her biggest feed of the day to set her up for the night ahead. As a result of milk depletion babies can be hard to settle in the evenings due to hunger, wanting to cluster feed and not wanting to be put down at bedtime. To combat this, express milk after the two morning feeds which will allow you to stagger the bedtime feed, introducing a bottle-feed after the bath. This is sometimes called the 'split feed' but I will call it the 'staggered feed': a short breastfeed of 10–15 minutes maximum (including winding) each side before the bath and a longer bottle-feed after the bath. The combination of the bath and staggered feed results in 4–8 hours of undisturbed sleep.

Expressing

Express within 20 minutes of finishing a feed to avoid stealing milk produced for the next feed. Express for 3–5 minutes on the first breast and then change sides. Repeat this a few times or, if using a double pump, start the stimulating mode and full cycle twice. Massaging your breasts while expressing will help to release the milk. Make sure you express for no more than 20 minutes (10 minutes on a double pump). You may not get very much milk at first but, don't despair, the amount will soon increase.

Keep your expressed breast milk in the fridge (it will keep for up to five days). If you are expressing more than you are using, which is normal, freeze the remaining milk daily (it will keep for up to six months in the freezer). This can then be used later on when weaning or if you ever need 'emergency' milk.

Playtime and stimulation

Toys, activity stations and setting up stimulating play areas, such as a play mat or baby chair, can make a huge difference to the length of awake time your baby can manage. Most babies are sleepy at the end of a feed and this is usually due to milk digestion rather than tiredness. Change your baby's nappy after a feed to encourage waking. Most babies also spring to life with the help of a black-and-white toy or picture.

During playtime, you will need to wind your baby several times, around 10–15 minutes apart, to alleviate any wind formed while digesting milk. This will also help your quest for a longer and happier playtime as a baby will naturally start to fall asleep as the wind builds while digesting.

Baby-led nights

Once you have established breastfeeding and your baby has regained her birth weight, is over 2.72kg (6lb) and is gaining weight, which should all happen at around Week 2, in contrast to your day routine you should let your baby wake of her own accord for feeds at night. This is where my technique differs from other baby experts who advise waking your baby on the dot for each feed day and night, or waking her for a 'dream feed' (a booster feed which is given before the parent would naturally go to bed). On my routine your nights are 'baby-led': if your baby is hungry, she will wake for a feed at night. By encouraging the majority of your baby's milk intake during the day, combined with the staggered feed and bottle at bedtime, there is no need to wake your baby for a dream feed. As your baby's day feeds and awake time increase over the weeks so will the length of time she sleeps at night, getting the much-needed rest to grow and thrive. As a result your baby will learn the difference between night and day very early on and night feeds will become efficient and short. You will also get the much-needed rest you need to recover and take care of your new baby.

When breastfeeding your baby will get into a routine much quicker than your breasts, which can leave you feeling full, uncomfortable and unable to last until your baby naturally wakes. Your breasts will also need extra stimulation to make up for the loss of stimulation from your baby as she sleeps longer at night at this early stage. Once your baby is waking past 1am, waking only once in the night or sleeping through the night, introduce a 'power pump' and express before you go to bed at 8–9pm. This will keep you comfortable and able to sleep until your baby naturally wakes, add extra stimulation to maintain a good milk supply and help you understand your milk supply and flow speed. As your milk supply increases overall, so will the amount of milk you express at this time. As the weeks go by your flow of milk will speed up. This express will show you how quickly your milk is released which will also help you to gauge how long it takes to drain your breast. Bear in mind that you will have much more milk at the start of the day.

Night feeds

Night waking and feeds should get gradually later through the night with the increase in your baby's awake time and milk intake during the day. The later your baby is waking through the night, the shorter the feed should be:

- 10pm–3am: 30 minutes (15 minutes each side), including winding, less if your baby wants
- 3am–4am: 20 minutes (10 minutes each side), including winding
- 4am–5am: 10 minutes (5 minutes each side), including winding and keep your baby swaddled. No nappy change (unless the nappy is dirty instead of wet)
- 5am–6am: No feed zone

Once your night feed has reached 4am, keep your baby swaddled. This will help keep the feed short, keep stimulation to a minimum and help her go back to sleep quickly after the feed. No nappy change is required unless it is dirty. Try using a larger size nappy for nights to accommodate a full night's sleep without changing. Make sure the nappy is fitted securely around the legs to prevent any leaks.

If your baby has slept all the way through until 5am or 6am, she has slept the majority of the night so feeding at this time will be stimulating and she will most likely want a breakfast feed, not a snack, to get back to sleep. Feeding at this time will dramatically interfere with the 7am feed which can have a knock-on effect on your whole day routine. If your baby wakes at this time, keep her swaddled and cuddle her back to sleep by holding her on your chest firmly (cover up any naked skin which will only frustrate and not calm your baby – use a muslin or pop a top on), patting her back and bottom, and breathing deeply. This is a form of the 'shush and hold' technique (see page 205). As a very last resort, let your baby suck on your finger which will calm and soothe her. Stay in your baby's bedroom or go back to your bed in the dark. Start your day at 6am and switch your routine to the four-hourly 6am routine that day. This is the only time of day I would advise letting your baby suck your finger or cuddling your baby back to sleep as I don't believe in babies sucking for comfort. It creates wind and has a negative effect on the morning feed.

When feeding your baby in the night, keep the lighting as low as possible so you can barely see and avoid talking or creating any stimulation. Feed your baby, wind her and then put her straight back to bed – this keeps the night-time feeds short and sweet so your baby is easy to settle. The more stimulation, the more awake your baby becomes, and the harder she will be to settle back to sleep. Swaddle your baby for the last 2–5 minutes of the breastfeed or the last 30ml (1oz) if giving a bottle, but where possible you should always breastfeed in the night even if you are mixed feeding. This will make for a calm transition from breast to bed.

Use the 'two-minute rule' for night waking. Allow a two-minute pause when your baby has woken to see if she settles back to sleep or is actually ready for a feed. Some babies grizzle, stretch and grunt for a while before waking properly, but please let your baby grizzle undisturbed. The chances are that she is still in 'sleep mode' with her eyes closed. If you rush in to feed your baby whenever you hear a cry or grizzle, you are not allowing her a chance to resettle. You may be starting a feed she is not ready for, only for her to wake again a few hours later when she is actually ready for milk. At night, babies go through lots of lighter periods of sleep and during those light periods they can twitch, turn, grizzle, and even cry a bit, but if left they will often go back to sleep.

Top tips for night feeding

- Keep your baby's room dark, using blackout blinds in the summer, and with no night light. Keep the camera monitor light covered as it will shine straight on to your baby's face. Once she has reached six weeks and wakes in the night, any light, albeit dim lighting, will stimulate her. Night lights can be used, if at all, much later on, at around six months plus.

- Keep night feeds in the same room as your baby sleeps in. Moving rooms, turning lights on and walking around are stimulating and will encourage waking. Practise short, dark, quiet feeds with no talking, phones or TV.

- Swaddle your baby at night until she is sleeping through the night for at least two weeks. If she wakes and the swaddle is loose or her arms have come out, this may be the only reason for waking and she will not be able to resettle with her arms waving around. Re-swaddle her, give her a cuddle and then pop her back to bed. Regardless of the reason for waking, a newborn will immediately think 'milk', so you may need to feed her if re-swaddling and resettling doesn't work. The swaddle technique is key to your baby settling! Tuck her into bed with no loose blankets. Babies feel secure, cuddled and sleep better if they are wrapped and firmly tucked in. This also helps to stop her waking due to the startle reflex. (See pages 198 and 202 for more advice on swaddling and tucking in.)

- Change your baby's nappy *before* night feeds. Changing her nappy after a feed will again stimulate her and encourage waking, making it more difficult for her to settle back to sleep.

- Night feeds should take no longer than 30 minutes, regardless of whether you are breast- or bottle-feeding. The idea is to change your baby, feed her and then put her back to bed quickly. The length and quantity of feeds should decrease the later your baby wakes (see page 64). This is to help phase out night feeds and to not interfere with the morning feed at 7am. The maximum for any one night feed is capped at 30 minutes or 120ml (4oz) from a bottle.

- Swaddle your baby for the last five minutes of the night feed and let her drift to sleep, winding her over your shoulder and then promptly putting her back to bed.

Room temperature

It's important to ensure that your baby does not overheat or get too cold. If a baby is cold she will wake; if she is too hot overheating becomes more of a danger. Everyone thinks that it's necessary to keep a baby warm with lots of layers, even putting on hats and mittens indoors, because babies are unable to regulate their own temperature. However, this is usually for the first few weeks of life until they start gaining weight and body fat. Even so, babies release heat through their skin so it's important to keep the room temperature above 18°C degrees at all times and not use hats indoors.

The ideal sleeping environment is a room temperature of 18–21°C with your baby dressed in a vest bodysuit, a Babygro or sleepsuit, a swaddle, roll pillows (if using) and one thick, stretchy blanket or two thinner blankets to tuck her in (see Chapter Thirteen for more on swaddling, sleep positions and tucking in). If in the summer months the temperature goes up, reduce the layers by removing the sleepsuit/Babygro first and use a thinner blanket to tuck your baby in. You should always keep the swaddle and a thin blanket, or even a large muslin, to tuck her in. If the room temperature reaches over 24°C look to cool it down by letting air in or using a fan, with the air flow not directly on your baby.

The ideal feeding/awake time temperature is 19–20°C. This is a little warmer than the sleeping temperature because I advise babies to be fed in a vest bodysuit, which means their arms and legs are exposed, but the room should be no hotter than 20°C as babies heat up while they are feeding and digesting.

Three-hourly Routine for Low Milk Supply

Weeks 2–3: Three-hourly Routine for Low Milk Supply	
6am	Start on left breast Feed for 30 minutes each side Express any remaining milk for 10–20 minutes Total awake and playtime (including feed): 1½–2 hours
7.30/8am	Nap
9am	Start on right breast Feed for 30 minutes each side Express any remaining milk for 10–20 minutes Total awake and playtime (including feed): 1½–2 hours
10.30/11am	Nap
12pm	Start on left breast Feed for 30 minutes each side Total awake and playtime (including feed): 1½ hours
1.30pm	Nap
3pm	Start on right breast Feed for 30 minutes each side Total awake and playtime (including feed): 1½ hours
4.30pm	Nap
6pm	Start on left breast Feed for 10–15 minutes each side (30 minutes maximum)
6.30pm	Bath (34–35°C)
6.45pm	Bottle-feed: expressed breast milk/formula 60–120ml (2–4oz), winding every 15–30ml (½–1oz)
7.15/7.30pm	Bedtime (swaddled)
During the night	Baby-led: feed for 15 minutes each side whenever your baby wakes Wait two minutes on waking to see if she resettles Change your baby's nappy before the feed Swaddle for the last 5 minutes of the feed

Notes on routine

- Milk intake and awake time will vary from baby to baby. Encourage a gradual increase of awake time until your baby reaches a full two hours at each day feed period, which should be easily obtained by around six weeks of age. Gradually increase your baby's daily milk intake until she reaches her own personal amount needed per feed to sleep through the night.
- For the first two morning feeds, express within 20 minutes of finishing the feed to avoid stealing milk produced for the next feed. With a three-hourly feeding routine it's important to express as close to the end of the feed as possible.
- This routine is not practical in the long-term but it can be used until your milk supply has increased. Move on to the 7pm–7am routine below as soon as you are able to.

The 7pm to 7am Sleeping Baby Routine

Once your baby is over 2.72kg (6lb) in weight, is gaining weight and is back to her birth weight, and your milk supply meets or is ahead of your baby's demand, you can move on to the 7pm to 7am Sleeping Baby Routine. The benefit of this routine is that your baby has more time to digest milk between each feed, which allows her stomach to empty between feeds and therefore for her to build an appetite to feed. At this stage your baby will also become more efficient at feeding and will take a gradually increasing amount of milk at each feed. On this routine you, as a mother, will have time for expressing, looking after yourself and resting between feeds, which can be more beneficial for your milk supply than feeding every three hours. This routine also introduces increased awake/playtime between feeds, which in turn encourages long sleep periods at night. Unlike other baby routines which state the ideal nap length, my routine focuses on your baby's awake time. Your baby's nap times will decrease as her awake time increases.

Breastfeeding on my 7pm–7am routine will take up to an hour in the first 6–8 weeks for all day feeds. Make sure you change sides when you have run out of milk on the first side (see page 48 for how to check your breasts for milk) or have fed your baby for 30 minutes (this includes winding). This is important, as it means your baby will suck for long enough to reach the rich 'hindmilk' that she needs to enable longer periods between feeds. If you swap breasts before your baby reaches the hindmilk, and therefore give two lots of foremilk, it will result in your baby 'snacking' as you will not have filled her up at each feed. This will also decrease your future milk supply as you will not have drained and stimulated your breasts to produce enough milk for the next feed. You should complete the feed (including winding) in one hour. Thirty minutes of active feeding and winding is long enough to drain one breast.

Low milk supply

If you are still struggling to get a good milk supply and your baby is not settling or maybe waking early for feeds due to hunger, you can top up with expressed milk or formula after the two morning feeds, keeping this top-up within the hour allocated for feeding. Breastfeed for 20 minutes on each side, or 30 minutes on one side and 15 on the other, then offer a top-up bottle, starting at 60ml (2oz) and increasing if needed. If you are finding that you are using both expressed milk and formula during the day, which includes your bedtime bottle, save the formula for the bedtime bottle where it will be most beneficial as it is heavier, takes longer to digest than breast milk and therefore will sustain your baby for longer, making it perfect for encouraging longer periods of sleep at night. If you are finding you need to top up regularly and are not happy with mixed feeding, there are a few things you can do to encourage a more productive milk supply (see page 29).

It can take weeks to get a tip-top milk supply and, while being in recovery with sleepless nights, your baby's demand can often be one step ahead of your milk supply. This routine allows you to get the milk supply benefits of a good night's sleep, as well as the extra stimulation of expressing, so your breasts don't lose out when your baby is sleeping for longer periods at night. If you are unable to meet your baby's daily demand and you want the routine to work in giving you a full night's sleep, then mixed feeding is the answer (see Chapter Six).

Breast milk test

If you want to investigate your milk supply once you are established, for instance because you are unsure of how much milk your baby is getting, you suspect you have a low milk supply, a fast let-down or initial flow, or you simply want to understand how your milk flow personally works for you, then the best way to do this is to express a full feed and offer your baby a bottle instead for that feed. You will need to express for 30 minutes on a double pump or 45–50 minutes on a single. Express 30 minutes before the feed is due and then again once you have finished feeding your baby so you are expressing as close to the feed time as possible. Ideally, get someone else to bottle-feed your baby while you express. Stop and switch sides once the flow stops or, if double pumping, stop and restart the stimulating mode once the flow has stopped.

If you want to check the speed of your milk flow, time how much milk you get in the first two minutes of expressing and record it, then again after another three minutes, which will give you the amount of milk you have expressed in five minutes. Then record how much milk your extract at five-minute intervals until you have finished. This should give you a good idea of when you should be breaking a feed to wind your baby. If your milk comes through quickly at first, then break to wind after two minutes on each breast and extend the amount of time between wind breaks as your milk flow slows down.

The best feed to do this 'breast milk test' is the mid-morning feed. You will have less milk at this time than at the first morning feed, but more than at the afternoon feed, so it will give you an average. The information you gain from this test, alongside the evening express, should give you a better understanding of your personal flow and milk supply. Be aware that your milk supply will go up and down for all sorts of reasons, such as your energy levels, activity, and your liquid and food intake. The speed of your milk flow will increase throughout the weeks as your milk thins and increases.

Be flexible

It may take weeks before you will be able to be consistent with the routine, depending on the night feed timings and morning waking. For instance, if your baby wakes at 6am, you would then be on a 6am, 10am, 2pm, 6pm routine for that day. The routine start time is bound to vary until your baby learns to sleep through the night. You can also change the routine to fit in with an appointment. For example, if you have an appointment at 11.30am, you could wake your baby earlier, changing the routine to feeding times of: 6.30am, 10am, 2pm, 6pm pre-bath feed, 6.30pm bath, 6.45pm bottle, 7/7.30pm bed. By ending the day at the same time you are able to get back on to your 7pm–7am routine the next day.

Alternative routine feed times

- 6am, 10am, 2pm, 6pm pre-bath feed, 6.30pm bath, 6.45pm bottle, 7.30pm bed
- 6.30am, 10/10.30am, 2/2.30pm, 6pm pre-bath feed, 6.30pm bath, 6.45pm bottle, 7.30pm bed
- 7am, 10.30/11am, 2.30pm, 6pm pre-bath feed, 6.30pm bath, 6.45pm bottle, 7.30pm bed

- 7/7.30am, 11am, 2.30/3pm, 6pm pre-bath feed, 6.30pm bath, 6.45pm bottle, 7.30pm bed
- 7.30am, 11.30am, 3pm, 6pm pre-bath feed, 6.30pm bath, 6.45pm bottle, 7.30pm bed

If you find changing the start time each morning confusing, you can wake your baby every morning at the same time no matter what happens at night. If you do this, make sure that the later you feed during the night, the smaller you make the feed (see page 64). Also the later your baby wakes the more stimulated she becomes so you need to keep feeding quick, quiet and dark with little to no stimulation.

It's a good idea to keep a baby routine diary. The easiest way to do this is to buy a diary that has one day per page. This helps you to see the pattern that is developing and work out your routine for each day.

Weeks 2–3: The 7pm to 7am Sleeping Baby Routine	
7am	Start on left breast Feed for 30 minutes each side Express any remaining milk within 20 minutes of finishing the feed Total awake and playtime (including feed): 1½–2 hours
8.30/9am	Nap
10.30/11am	Start on right breast Feed for 30 minutes each side Express any remaining milk within 20 minutes of finishing the feed Total awake and playtime (including feed): 1½–2 hours
12/1pm	Nap

2.30pm	Start on left breast Feed for 30 minutes each side Total awake and playtime (including feed): 1½–2 hours
4/4.30pm	Nap
6pm	Start on right breast Feed for 10–15 minutes each side (30 minutes maximum)
6.30pm	Bath (34–35°C)
6.45pm	Bottle-feed: expressed breast milk/formula 60–150ml (2–5oz)
7/7.30pm	Bedtime (swaddled)
8/9pm	Express once your baby is regularly waking past 1am or 2am
During the night	Baby-led: for 10–15 minutes each side maximum whenever your baby wakes Wait two minutes on waking to see if she resettles Change your baby's nappy before the feed Swaddle for the last 5 minutes of the feed

Notes on routine

- Milk intake and awake time will vary from baby to baby. Encourage a gradual increase of awake time until your baby reaches a full two hours at each day feed period, which should be easily obtained by around six weeks of age. Gradually increase your baby's daily milk intake until she reaches her own personal amount needed per feed to sleep through the night.
- Day feeds take up to an hour, including winding; night feeds take up to 30 minutes, including winding.
- Keep a diary to keep track of progress.
- Wake your baby 10–15 minutes before each day feed. All day feeds and the bedtime bottle-feed are to be fed

in just a vest bodysuit to help keep your baby cool while feeding.

- The perfect room temperature for feeding is 19–20°C.
- Your baby's awake time is counted from the start of a feed, not the 10–15 minutes used to wake her before a feed.
- Change your baby's nappy *after* feeding during the daytime to help wake her for playtime. Babies usually fill their nappies while feeding. If you need to change your baby's nappy before the feed then also change after the feed.
- Change your baby's nappy before feeding during the night-time. This avoids stimulation before settling. If she wakes more than once, change her nappy at the first waking only unless she has a dirty nappy. When your baby is sleeping through the night, try using a larger size nappy for nights to accommodate a full night's sleep without changing. Make sure the nappy is fitted securely around the legs to prevent any leaks.
- The nights are baby-led, which means you should let your baby wake naturally for the night feeds. Use the two-minute rule with night waking before reacting to make sure your baby has in fact woken for a feed. Babies wake often during the night and resettle themselves back to sleep.
- Go to bed early to ensure you get enough sleep. Your milk supply will thank you for it, as will your body and mental health. Your body first uses energy to recover from giving birth, second for daily activity and last for lactation. A skin-on-skin nap during the day with your new baby will certainly boost your milk supply and your well-being, and is a beautiful bonding experience.
- Keep night feeds short and sweet (10–15 minutes each side). Feed in a dark room in silence. The later your baby wakes the less time should be spent feeding. The longer between feeds the more efficient your baby will feed with the more free-flowing milk you will have.

- Your newborn should be able to sleep at least 4–5 hours between feeds at night. If she doesn't, you need to work out why this is. Increase the length of her daytime play-time, increase her milk intake and encourage active feeding with no comfort sucking or snoozing during feeds.
- Before swapping breasts during a feed check your breasts for milk (see page 48). Your baby may have drained the breast in 20 minutes. Swap breasts when the first is completely empty or after 30 minutes.
- If you are producing milk like a prize dairy cow, you may need to swap breasts before it looks like you have 'run out' since your baby may refuse to suck when the milk flow slows. She would have reached the hindmilk but, being flow sensitive, may not be able to or be interested in completely draining your breast. You also need to be stim-ulating both breasts equally. Many mothers with fast-flowing milk have lazy feeders as their babies don't have to suck hard to get the hindmilk. Remember to start on alternate breasts at each feed.
- Swaddle your newborn when you put her to bed at night-time – she will sleep for longer with a swaddle as it stops her waking herself with the startle reflex and she will feel cuddled and secure. Try not to use the swaddle but tuck her in tight around the shoulders during daytime naps. If you are starting this routine at a later stage and are finding daytime naps unsettled, swaddle your baby for the day naps as well as during the night. I would say that 75 per cent of the babies in my care need to be swaddled during the day as well as the night, but for recognising the difference between night and day and getting your baby used to sleeping without the swaddle I would always try not using the swaddle during the day.

Chapter Five

Week 4 Onwards

At Weeks 4–6 the consistency of your breast milk thins. Think of your milk starting out as cream (colostrum), changing to full-fat milk, then to semi-skimmed and then to skimmed by four months. As this happens the flow of your milk dramatically speeds up which can speed up the whole feeding process. When this happens you may need to cut down the length of time you breastfeed your baby for the pre-bath feed. Day feeds may become shorter as your baby can drain your breast in less time, but I would always allow an hour to make sure he is full until he is sleeping through the night.

You may have only one night waking at this stage, or your baby may even be sleeping through the night. When this happens, express both breasts before you go to bed at 8–9pm. It is unrealistic to think your breasts can supply enough milk in the 12-hour day period and be inactive at night, so expressing at this time of the day helps maintain a good milk supply and aids your comfort through the night.

The longer your baby sleeps through the night the more a solid habit of sleeping becomes, which also coincides with unsettled day naps. Again, it is unrealistic to expect your baby to sleep so well at night, so early on, and also have three solid naps in the day. You are still teaching your baby the difference between night and day, and to sleep at night and decreasingly sleep during the day. To help combat this unsettled period, extend your baby's playtime by 10–15 minutes, adjust his feed times to accommodate early waking during the day or start swaddling him for the daytime naps. It's also important to understand that consistency of solid night sleeping will be down to meeting your baby's needs during the day.

Be flexible

Babies have 'mini growth spurts' on a weekly basis and the routine won't always go to plan. Just allow the routine to be flexible. Continue to encourage awake time and make sure your baby is full at each feed to ensure a good night-time sleep. If at this stage you are getting frequent night wakings or your baby is unsettled between feeds then check:

- Your milk supply and baby's intake (increase his milk intake at the bedtime bottle)
- That you are winding your baby effectively
- That he has long enough awake time between feeds
- Your baby's sleep position (see page 199)

The routine timings are interchangeable as they all end the day at the same time. Sticking to the same timings will help set your baby's body clock but there is no reason why you can't move from one routine to another every so often, depending on night and morning wakings or to simply plan around appointments and activities. Below are some alternative routine feed timings:

- 6am, 10am, 2pm, 6pm pre-bath feed, 6.30pm bath, 6.45pm bottle, 7.30/8pm bed
- 6.30am, 10/10.30am, 2/2.30pm, 6pm pre-bath feed, 6.30pm bath, 6.45pm bottle, 7.30/8pm bed
- 7am, 10.30/11am, 2.30pm, 6pm pre-bath feed, 6.30pm bath, 6.45pm bottle, 7.30/8pm bed

- 7/7.30am, 11am, 2.30/3pm, 6pm pre-bath feed, 6.30pm bath, 6.45pm bottle, 7.30/8pm bed
- 7.30am, 11.30am, 3pm, 6pm pre-bath feed, 6.30pm bath, 6.45pm bottle, 7.30/8pm bed

So you can see how flexible your routine can be to suit your baby's sleep needs.

Once your baby is sleeping through the night and has reached his maximum milk intake, you will need to be consistent with your routine to maintain results. Your routine from Weeks 8–10 should start to require less effort as feeds speed up as your baby's gut has matured and he now starts to become self-winding, is able to stay awake with ease, settles himself for naps and starts being able to stay awake in motion, which takes all restrictions out of your previous daily routine. From Weeks 10–12 your baby's rate of growth will have started to slow a little and his appetite will plateau. Once established and out of the newborn stage, the longer your baby sleeps through the night the more flexible the routine becomes as his appetite will go up and down slightly, he sleeps less during the day and is able to wait happily for feeds. Allow your routine to become more flexible with milk intake and timings, but do keep to the bedtime routine to keep consistency with bedtime and sleeping through the night.

Once your baby is sleeping through the night change the starting breast every morning. You will now have four breast-feeds per day and, unless you start each day on the opposite breast, you will be starting each feed with the same starter breast and the other breast may not get the same stimulation.

Playtime and stimulation

By now you should really be enjoying playtime with your baby and starting to get a few smiles. Your baby may start to track and follow so using a cot mobile for awake time and toys dangling from the arches of a play mat may start to hold interest, but most babies are still more interested in black-and-white images and their parents' faces. A baby's attention span shortens as the weeks go by with the ability to see at a distance and follow movement, and static black-and-white toys will no longer offer the same entertainment by Weeks 6–8. Your baby may decide that the best place to be is with you, being carried around and complaining about being put down to play. It is important, however, that he still has some time playing on his own and is not being picked up and put down every few minutes when he grizzles. It will only make for a more demanding and insecure baby who is less able to play by himself. Whenever your baby cries to be picked up, use your voice to soothe him, rotate his toys, try tummy time or move him to a different area of the house – perhaps in his chair where he can watch you. Simply holding your baby's feet can give him security of your touch and will often calm and distract. Toys with squeaky and rustle sounds, such as the Lamaze Jacques the Peacock, are also a big favourite at this time.

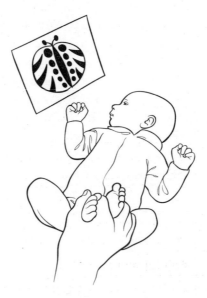

Holding feet to reassure and calm baby during playtime

The first half of playtime is the best time for self-play, so put your baby down to play on a play mat while you express and look after yourself. Ensure you don't give your baby tummy time sooner than 30 minutes after a feed, as you need to allow time for digestion. The end of the playtime, as your baby starts to get tired and grumpy and needs distracting, can be reserved for one-on-one chat time with you. Finally enjoy a cuddle before his nap. Remember to check for wind during your baby's playtime. Wind is formed while digesting milk and can be the cause of grizzles or falling asleep during playtime. Most newborns therefore need to burp a few times before going down for a nap.

Week 4 Onwards: The 7pm to 7am Sleeping Baby Routine	
7am	Start on left breast Feed for 25–30 minutes each side Express any remaining milk Total awake and playtime (including feed): 2–2¼ hours
9am/9.15am	Nap
10.30/11am	Start on right breast Feed for 25–30 minutes each side Express any remaining milk Total awake and playtime (including feed): 2–2¼ hours
12.30/1.15pm	Nap
2.30/3pm	Start on left breast Feed for 25–30 minutes each side Total awake and playtime (including feed): 2 hours
4.30/5pm	Nap
6pm	Start on right breast Feed for 5–10 minutes each side
6.30pm	Bath (34–35°C)
6.45/7pm	Bottle-feed: expressed breast milk/formula 180–260ml (6–9oz)

7/7.30pm	Bedtime (swaddled)
During the night	12am–3am: 15 minutes on each side 3am–4am: 10 minutes on each side 4am–5am: 15 minutes total, keep baby swaddled 5am–6am: No feed zone

Notes on routine

- Milk intake and awake time will vary from baby to baby. Encourage a gradual increase of awake time until your baby reaches a full two hours at each day feed period, which should be easily obtained by around six weeks of age. Gradually increase your baby's daily milk intake until he reaches his own personal amount needed per feed to sleep through the night. Only increase his awake time to 2¼ hours if he is waking early for feeds and you feel he needs less sleep during the day. This wouldn't normally happen until he is over six weeks of age. There is no need to extend his awake time if he is sleeping well day and night.

- At around six weeks of age your baby will have a major growth spurt, at which time he may become very hungry and very tired. Try topping up after feeds if your baby is still hungry coming off the breast and keep solid awake time where possible. You want your baby to take any extra sleep he needs to grow at night.

- Your baby will also be developing his personality and will start to have an opinion on what he wants to do at this age. He is also easily distracted, which you can use in a positive way to keep to the routine. The 10–15 minutes waking before each feed can now be used for chats and play before moving on to a quiet and focused feed. Now your baby is interactive he will want to smile and chat with you once the edge is taken off his appetite so try to exhaust this before the feed.

- From Weeks 6–8 your baby may be happy to wait for feeds making early waking and short naps less of an issue to stay on track with your routine. The routine becomes much more flexible at this stage with regards to day naps.
- As your baby's attention span shortens from Week 8, you will need more interactive toys, such as a moving mobile.
- Even if your baby is still having an afternoon nap, he may be tired and grizzly at the end of the day no matter how much sleep he has had. This is normal throughout a child's life. Much as we, as adults, get tired towards the end of the day, it's the same for babies and children.
- If your baby is feeding well, weighs over 4.08kg (9lb) and is awake for two hours at each daytime feed period and drinking over 180ml (6oz) at his bedtime bottle, he could well be sleeping through the night by six weeks, or even earlier. He may be sleeping through but waking early, around 6am. If this is the case, you may need to adjust your routine for a while, to the 6am four-hourly routine, until he is able to sleep until 7am.

This routine now continues until weaning (at around 4–6 months), bearing in mind that the daytime sleeps will continue to get lighter as your baby sleeps more heavily at night. This is especially true of the afternoon nap, which reduces to 20 minutes in some cases and this is the first nap that your baby will drop. When this happens, it is a good idea to alter the afternoon routine and only have a three-hour gap between the last two feeds of the day. Change the routine feed timings to: 7am, 11am, 3pm, 6pm pre-bath feed, 6.30pm bath, 6.45pm bottle. You want to focus on a solid long midday nap. If you find your baby is unsettled on his second nap of the day, reduce his morning nap to ensure a longer more solid nap at lunch, which will benefit your baby's temperament when he starts dropping the afternoon nap.

Implementing a Routine at a Later Stage

Many of you will be reading this book because you have run into problems with on-demand feeding and now want to try to encourage your baby into a routine. The flexibility of my routine makes this quite simple. If your baby is snacking and taking small quantities of milk frequently, he will need to increase his milk intake gradually and you will need to work on increasing your milk supply. The greater your baby's appetite and the greater his milk intake, the longer the milk intake will sustain him between feeds.

Under six weeks of age, start with the three-hourly routine for the first few days to a week to help maintain enough milk intake during the day and allow time for your breasts to increase their supply at each feed. Then move on to the 3½-hourly routine, aiming for the 7pm–7am routine within two weeks of starting a routine, which will allow for bigger feeds and increased awake time. It may take a while for your baby to get used to taking more milk at each feed if he is currently used to snacking. If he is sleeping a great deal in the day, wake him for feeds and try to keep him awake afterwards for as long as you can, aiming for two hours at each feed period and building the routine gradually. Do not let him go more than four hours between feeds during the day. Conversely, at night your baby should not be fed more often than four-hourly. Split the bedtime feed with a bath, as suggested, to increase his milk intake before bed. The case study below shows how quickly you can turn things round from chaos to calm.

Jessica and Lucy (four weeks old)

Jessica contacted me on a Monday needing help with her four-week-old baby, Lucy. Lucy weighed 4.59kg (10lb 2oz) and was feeding every 2–3 hours, day and night. Jessica had trouble with thrush on her nipples and Lucy would not latch on to the breast properly, so Jessica was expressing her breast milk and Lucy was taking about 90ml (3oz) per feed. Lucy was sleeping well in the day, but was awake all night. She was not having any playtime and was being put straight to bed after each feed. Although she was having a bath at 6.30pm, Lucy did not have a feed afterwards but was being put straight to sleep.

Monday

I could see that Lucy was not taking enough milk at each feed so I advised Jessica to increase her bottle to 120–150ml (4–5oz) per feed during daytime feeds and decrease the night feeds to a maximum of 90ml (3oz). I also recommended reducing the size of the feed before her bath to a maximum of 60ml (2oz) and introducing a larger feed after the bath. I asked Jessica to try to keep Lucy awake after the daytime feeds so that she was awake for 1½–2 hours at each feed period, timed from the start of each feed. I suggested the following routine:

7am	150ml (5oz) bottle of expressed breast milk
	Awake for 1½–2 hours
10.30am	120–150ml (4–5oz) bottle of expressed breast milk
	Awake for 1½–2 hours
2/2.30pm	120–150ml (4–5oz) bottle of expressed breast milk
	Awake for 1½–2 hours
5.30/6pm	60ml (2oz) bottle of expressed breast milk
6/6.30pm	Bath
6.30/7pm	120–150ml (4–5oz) bottle of expressed breast milk or formula
	Awake for 1½–2 hours (including feeds and bath)
7/7.30pm	Bed

Night feeds 4 hours minimum apart, 90ml (3oz) bottle of expressed breast milk, 30 minutes maximum

Thursday

Jessica telephoned to report a great improvement. She was very happy that the routine had fallen into place quite quickly, although it had taken Lucy a couple of days to take a full 120–150ml (4–5oz) at each feed. Once Jessica had increased intervals between feeds to every 3½ hours, it was easier to get Lucy to take 150ml (5oz). Jessica had found it hard to keep up with expressing her milk so she was supplementing with formula at the bedtime bottle. Lucy was still having two feeds at night which were also formula (90ml/3oz at 11pm and 3am). However, Lucy was hard to settle after these feeds and was awake for hours at a time. I discovered that, when Lucy woke at night, Jessica was in the habit of getting Lucy up and taking her downstairs to prepare the bottle. I advised Jessica that she should stop using formula for the night feeds, and give no more than 90ml (3oz) of expressed breast milk for each of these night feeds as expressed milk makes for a lighter meal than formula. Instead, she should use formula as needed during the day and give only formula at the staggered bedtime feed. At night, Lucy should not be taken downstairs. Jessica should prepare the night-time bottles and then go in to Lucy so she could go straight from cot to bottle, be winded well and then straight back to bed. Lucy should have minimal stimulation at night – keep the lights low, no talking and only change her nappy before a night feed and only if dirty on the second night feed. Jessica had also mentioned that Lucy was not happy during playtime but had not been given any toys or pictures to look at. I suggested making some simple black-and-white pictures for Lucy to help entertain her.

I also felt Jessica could increase the daytime feeds to 180ml (6oz). The increase of milk would discourage night waking and encourage the first night feed gradually getting later through the night, waking between 3am and 5am. Whatever time Lucy woke, Jessica should be sure to start the day at 7am. To help Lucy to stay awake after her daytime feeds, I recommended various play options – a play mat, using black-and-white toys, putting Lucy down to play somewhere where she could see Jessica (for example, in her baby chair), having tummy time and having one-on-one chat time. I emphasised how important it was to keep Lucy awake for 1½–2 hours in the daytime.

The following Monday

Jessica rang me absolutely thrilled. Lucy was only waking briefly at around 11pm, but was resettling herself, and then again for a feed between 3am and 4am. She was taking a quick feed of 20 minutes and going straight back to sleep. Lucy was now taking 150–180ml (5–6oz) at day feeds and 180–200ml (6–7oz) of formula before bed and was having good awake time in the day.

My final advice was to remember not to jump to Lucy's every cry and to leave her for two minutes before going to her at night, as I felt she was probably waking out of habit, especially as she was taking 180–200ml (6–7oz) before bed. If Lucy grizzled or did 'start–stop' shouting, so not properly crying at night, I advised Jessica to leave her a little longer than two minutes to see if she settled herself. When stop–start crying a baby is half asleep and not fully awake. Jumping to help too quickly will often stimulate her awake rather than resettle her. Also moving forwards with the routine, I advised Jessica to increase Lucy's milk intake until she was sleeping through the night. In just one week, Lucy went from being awake most of the night to waking only briefly for a short feed. It might take a little longer for

Lucy to sleep through the night than it would have done if Jessica had started the routine at birth, but I felt that, in another month, Lucy should be sleeping through the night.

Months 4–6 Onwards

My routine will take you up to the weaning stage. The only differences with the routine between the newborn stage and the now established baby stage are:

1. *The length of sleep needed during the day is reduced.* Your baby may have already dropped his afternoon nap or be having a very short one. The length of sleep a baby needs during the day varies from baby to baby, but the general focus should be on a longer lunchtime nap of 1½–2 hours. Keeping this nap in your baby's cot as much as possible, and therefore providing the right sleeping environment, will help keep this nap solid. This lunchtime nap will stay part of your child's routine until he is around three years old. If for any reason your baby's lunchtime nap is unsettled, extend his morning awake time to 2½–3 hours and reduce his morning nap to increase the length of sleep he has over the middle of the day, which in turn will help to reduce and phase out the afternoon nap. The morning nap should be 30–60 minutes long.

   Once your baby has dropped his afternoon nap, you might find that you need to bring the pre-bath feed earlier to 5.30pm, but still keep to the bath time of 6.30pm. The post-bath bottle should now be super-efficient and your baby should be going to bed nearer to 7pm.

2. *Sleep position.* Your baby will now be sleeping in a cot and possibly moving around and sleeping in a sleeping bag. Keep your baby tucked in for as long as he is not moving. Babies who move around and roll in their cot too

early often get stuck in positions and then wake and cry out for help to move them back.

3. *Your routine is now much more flexible* and you are able to feed your baby while out and about. Your baby can now stay awake in motion so you are no longer restricted to only going out at nap times, and his awake and playtimes can often be on the move or during activities such as meeting friends or baby groups.

4. *Feed times and quantities can be flexible* as your baby's appetite goes up and down, but don't change your baby's bath and bottle times as it is important to be consistent with bedtime. This part of the routine will not change until your baby is a child and his bedtime bottle is replaced with story time. When breastfeeding, by Months 3–4 the flow of your milk speeds up dramatically and your baby is now self-winding and can take much more milk between burping. This speeds up the length of time spent feeding to 30–40 minutes. If your baby is not yet sleeping through the night, still allow an hour for each day feed.

Weaning

Though the blanket advice from the Department of Health is to wean your baby at six months (26 weeks) of age, I do things a little differently and, if necessary, wean babies on to solid food ever so slowly from four months. Research evidence has proven that babies are digestively ready to be weaned on to solid food between four and six months, but, for some reason, the government advice has been set at six months. Waiting until six months with a baby who is ready to be weaned from four months will cause night waking, disruptive days and frustration, which may be mistaken for teething which occurs at around the same time. Starting solids as soon as you see the signs that your baby is ready (see below) means that you are able to take a slower approach to introducing solid food, which is, of course, better for your baby's digestion.

As babies get older, they have much more of an opinion on everything, including what goes into their mouths. There is certainly a difference between a baby of four months and a baby of six months in this respect. Starting weaning at six months often means it can be a stressful process as it's a rush to get your baby fully weaned as quickly as possible. A baby who is actually ready for food from four months can spend two weeks simply introducing a few spoons at one meal a day, and this gives you time to build the quantities. For those of you with babies who are not ready to wean until 5–6 months, enjoy the ease of milk feeding as it all gets a bit messy from here on in!

Below are signs to look out for when deciding if your baby is ready to be weaned:

- *Your baby starts waking at night having slept through for the last month or so.* He wakes due to hunger but is not interested in upping his milk intake during the day. At around four months some babies can lose interest in their milk. Night waking is believed to be the result of a growth spurt, but in my experience a growth spurt often means a baby is more hungry or sleeps more, so if your baby is waking having slept through for months, it makes sense that his food intake should be the first thing to address. Some mothers who are breastfeeding look to introduce formula as a stopgap to satisfy their baby until they are ready to start weaning.
- *Your baby is very interested in watching you eat* and often dribbles while watching you and will look like he is chewing. This is not the same as your baby chewing on his hands, as all babies do this as soon as they are able to and while teething.
- *Your baby can hold his own head up and sit when supported.*
- *Your baby dramatically goes off his milk or is no longer satisfied with his milk intake during the day.* Yes, milk

has more calories than puréed carrot but it is liquid and won't sustain your baby as long as solid food will. It takes weeks to build the amount of solid food a baby takes, so weaning is initially a supplement to your baby's milk.

- *Your baby can swallow.* Babies who aren't yet ready to be weaned will still have the tongue thrust reflex, which pushes food out of their mouths before swallowing.

Please talk to your health visitor or GP for advice if you feel your baby is ready to be introduced to solid food before six months.

In short ...

- The routine is based on feeding every 3–4 hours, timed from the start of each feed, during the day.
- During feeding it is important to encourage your baby not to fall asleep on the breast but to feed efficiently.
- You may need to wake your baby for feeds in the daytime, but not at night.
- The staggered feed before bed is split with bath time, ensuring that your baby is well fed before he goes to sleep.
- During the day, playtime and stimulation after each feed will encourage your baby to be more awake in the daytime and sleep at night.
- Night-time feeds are smaller and all stimulation should be avoided so that your baby is encouraged to be sleepier at night-time.
- Try to feed at intervals of four hours or more at night.
- If you are mixed feeding (both breast milk and formula – see Chapter Six), only use formula during the day not at night. The most beneficial time for formula is the bedtime bottle. Keep enough breast milk for the night feeds and then for the afternoon feed.

- As your baby sleeps better at night, his daytime naps may become lighter and shorter.
- Some days might not go according to plan, for instance during growth spurts, when the routine will not work so well. Don't worry – just be flexible and keep encouraging good habits. Your baby is not a robot and will always throw something new into the mix.
- Your baby's digestion is key to a settled comfortable baby: less wind + more milk = sleeping longer at night (see Chapter One).

Chapter Six

Mixed Feeding

The mixed feeding routine is for breastfeeding mothers with a low milk supply or if tandem feeding twins, and is right for you if you:

- want to give your baby as much breast milk as possible while filling her up at each feed in order for her to sleep through the night;
- want to supplement temporarily while increasing your milk supply; or
- simply want the best of both, to take the pressure off breastfeeding.

If you are tandem feeding twins, see Chapter Ten and the routine table on page 147 for specific timings and quantities for twins. While it's true that breast milk is best for your baby, often breastfeeding mothers are forever chasing their growing baby's appetite and need to supplement. Your milk supply is personal to you and, although there are many ways to increase your supply (see page 29), the reality is that you might not be able to supply enough milk to satisfy your baby and help her sleep through the night at the same time. To exclusively breastfeed you may need to feed every 2–3 hours day and night. If that's not for you then mixed feeding is the answer by giving your baby as much breast milk as possible and then topping her up with expressed breast milk and/or formula.

When mixed feeding with a combination of breast and bottle, the breastfeed must be given first and then top up with a bottle straight after, not the other way round. The bottle has an easier and often faster flow so offering the bottle first would result in less breast stimulation and a decreasing milk supply. Choosing to give only the breast or bottle at any one feed will have the same effect on your milk supply.

The quantity of milk given as a top-up will, of course, vary depending on how much milk your breasts are producing. If your baby takes the top-up easily after the breastfeed then try increasing the quantity of the top-up bottle. Make sure your breastfeed is active (see page 48), otherwise you could find your baby relies on the bottle for the bulk of her feed.

Once your baby is sleeping through the night and has reached her maximum milk intake, you will need to be consistent with your routine to maintain results. Your routine from Weeks 8–10 should start to require little effort as feeds speed up as your baby's gut has matured and she now starts to become self-winding, is able to stay awake with ease, settles herself for naps and starts being able to stay awake in motion, which takes all restrictions out of your previous daily routine. From Weeks 10–12 your baby's rate of growth will have started to slow a little and her appetite will plateau. The longer your baby sleeps through the night the more flexible your routine and feeds become as her appetite will go up and down slightly by 30–60ml (1–2oz) per feed. Try and keep the bedtime bottle consistent.

Weeks 3–5: Mixed Feeding Routine to Supplement Breastfeeding	
7am	Start on left breast Breastfeed for 40 minutes (20 minutes each side) + 30–90ml (1–3oz) formula Express any remaining milk Total awake and playtime (including feed): 1½–2 hours

8.30/9am	Nap
10.30/11am	Start on right breast Breastfeed for 40 minutes (20 minutes each side) + 60–90ml (2–3oz) expressed breast milk/formula Express any remaining milk Total awake and playtime (including feed): 1½–2 hours
12/1pm	Nap
2.30pm	Start on left breast Breastfeed for 30–40 minutes (15–20 minutes each side) + 60–90ml (2–3oz) expressed breast milk/formula Total awake and playtime (including feed): 1½–2 hours
4/4.30pm	Nap
6pm	Start on right breast Breastfeed for 20–30 minutes (10–15 minutes each side maximum)
6.30pm	Bath (34–35°C)
6.45pm	Bottle-feed 120–180ml (4–6oz) formula
7.15/8pm	Bedtime (swaddled)
8/9.30pm	Express once your baby is regularly waking past 1am and you are breastfeeding
During the night	11pm–3am: 90–120ml (3–4oz) bottle maximum or breastfeed for 15 minutes each side 3am–4am: 90ml (3oz) bottle maximum or breastfeed for 10 minutes each side 4am–5am: 60–90ml (2–3oz) bottle maximum or breastfeed for 10–15 minutes total, keep baby swaddled 5am–6am: No feed zone Wind every 30ml (1oz) or 5 minutes on breast

Notes on routine

- Milk intake and awake time will vary from baby to baby.
  Encourage a gradual increase of awake time until your
  baby reaches a full two hours at each day feed period,

which should be easily obtained by around six weeks of age. Gradually increase your baby's daily milk intake until she reaches her own personal amount needed per feed to sleep through the night.

- The above routine is a mixed feeding routine to supplement breastfeeding with the main focus being on breastfeeding, maintaining and encouraging a good milk supply by active stimulation and expressing while mixed feeding. This is time-consuming and a lot of work. Make sure the breast pump is ready to use and bottle made and ready before starting the breastfeed. The length of time for breastfeeding is slightly different for twins – please see Chapter Ten.

- The bulk of feeds are breast milk with top-ups to make sure your baby is full at each feed. The amount needed to top up will depend on your supply. Your milk supply depletes throughout the day so top-ups will naturally increase throughout the day, with the bedtime bottle, as with all the routines, being the largest feed of the day.

- When combining expressed breast milk and formula for the top-up bottles, it's important to give your baby formula at the right time of day to help in your quest for a full night's sleep. Breast milk is lighter, often less sustaining and digests quicker than formula, so use expressed breast milk for night feeds and the afternoon top-up, with any left over for the mid-morning feed. You are trying to encourage less filling feeds at night and giving a lighter feed at the afternoon feed will encourage a bigger appetite for the most important feed of the day, which is the bedtime feed. Formula will sustain your baby for longer so should therefore be given at the post-bath, bedtime bottle and then, if needed, the first morning feed.

- Try to keep day feeds to a maximum of one hour. This allows enough time for your baby's stomach to empty between feeds and for her to build an appetite before the next feed. It also encourages efficient feeding. Have your top-up bottles ready before starting the breastfeed. Cap your breastfeed at 45 minutes, leaving 15 minutes for the top-up. For twins, feed for 30 minutes maximum, one breast each, and then top up. You will be giving half the feed through a bottle so you will need more time to do so, also a baby should be able to drain a breast in 30 minutes including winding time.

- Expressing between 8pm and 9.30pm helps you to get to know your breasts, your flow speed and supply. This express also helps to maintain your supply and keeps you comfortable until your baby, or babies, naturally wakes later in the night. Add in this additional express when the first night feed is after 1am.

- Between four and six weeks your milk thins and the flow speeds up. You should see the difference when you squeeze down through the nipple. Instead of beading and drops you will now spray milk or large drips. The faster your flow the quicker your baby can drain your breasts if actively sucking. When this happens, reduce the time spent breastfeeding to 30–40 minutes in total, 20 minutes when feeding twins, and then top up. Reduce the pre-bath feed to 5–10 minutes each side.

- Allow your routine to become more flexible with milk intake and timings once your baby is sleeping through the night solidly for a few weeks, and more so when you reach the baby stage from 12 weeks old. However, do keep to the bedtime routine to keep consistency with bedtime and sleeping through the night.

PART TWO

Bottle-feeding

Chapter Seven

Bottle-feeding: the Basics

B ottle-feeding can make easy work of implementing a routine. Yes, breastfeeding is best for baby but for some mothers this simply isn't an option. Bottle-feeding allows you to be aware of your baby's milk intake and have control over the quantities more accurately, day and night. Breast milk is naturally easier to digest than formula, but with a wide range of specialist formulas these days, you can easily find a formula that suits your baby's digestion.

Which Formula?

My go-to formula milk is Aptamil. Of the cow's milk formulas, it has the least amount of lactose which is the sugar that some babies find hard to digest. Organic formulas, such as HiPP, produced by grass-fed cows, are also very popular but are not always as organic as the advertising suggests, and I have found that babies drinking this specific organic formula have increased vomiting. Stage 2 formulas are a gimmick and your baby can stay on Stage 1 until he is old enough to drink cow's milk (at one year). Aptamil Hungry Infant Milk is a good addition for the bedtime feed if you are having trouble filling your baby up for the night. However, I would advise not to give your baby this formula in his first month of life. Give your baby an opportunity to increase his milk intake naturally before using this trick later on if your normal formula is not doing the job. Hungry milk has the same amount of calories, but will sustain your baby for longer. There seems to be a trend nowadays of buying ready-made formula, but please use the powdered milk. As you might expect, ready-made formula has far more preservatives in it – it is essentially a ready meal for babies.

Formulas have come a long way in the last 10 years and are nutritionally high-tech with most brands offering alternative formulas for babies with a gut sensitivity. A better under-standing of reflux, dairy intolerance and newborn immature gut issues has led to leading brands introducing their own specialist formulas. Only if your baby is diagnosed with a gut issue by a specialist would he be prescribed a formula such as Nutramigen, Enfamil or Neocate. These formulas smell bad, taste sour and have a thinner consistency to regular formula causing other feeding issues, such as affecting the flow of milk and rejection due to the unpleasant taste.

Most babies have some kind of digestive issue simply due to their immature gut and being unable to self-wind in the first 8–12 weeks of life. A gut issue like reflux tends to creep in at around Weeks 3–6 with a baby's increased milk intake. If your baby is unhappy feeding or bloats during feeds, regardless of winding every 15–30ml (½–1oz), try switching to a lactose-free formula. If this doesn't help, see your GP who will advise on dairy-free options.

For formula-fed babies and babies born by C-section, I rec-ommend giving a daily dose of probiotics to help boost good gut bacteria and their immune system. Don't go cheap on this – use high-quality otherwise the benefits might be minimal (see page 12).

Which Bottle?

There are so many options of bottles and teats on the market and they offer anything from the promise of colic relief and wind-reducing valves, to 'closer to breastfeeding' and different speed teats. I've found many of their selling points to be gimmicks. The wind-reducing valves rarely work and often make the bottles leak. What they tend to do is actually slow the milk flow which in itself can reduce wind if your baby has a strong suck and gulps their milk. However, they can also create wind if your baby has a weak suck as the flow is too slow and the baby is sucking with very little reward, often taking in more air than milk. Only use a bottle such as Dr Brown's if your baby has a strong suck and excess wind.

Wind-reducing while feeding is more about finding the right flow and shape of teat for your baby's mouth and suck. Your baby could have a weak or strong suck which will inevitably change as he grows. A newborn will need to start with a size one, slow flow teat of which the speed will vary between brands. If your baby has a soft suck then a faster speed slow flow teat like MAM will work well and has a great shape to fit perfectly in your baby's mouth. A baby with a strong suck may find this teat too fast and be better suited to a Dr Brown's or Avent Classic teat. I tend to mix and match bottles and teats as I have not yet found a bottle and teat combination that I like. There are three teats that fit on an Avent Classic bottle: the Avent Classic teat, MAM teat and Dr Brown's teat. Here you have one bottle and three different options of flow and shape. You must buy the Classic style bottle for this combination. My go-to teat is the MAM to start with as it really is the perfect shape. However, it is easily compressed by a strong suck. If this happens, you will need to make sure your baby's mouth comes up to the curve of the teat, twist the teat to delatch and inflate the teat again. Regardless of this little issue with the teat, it is still my favourite teat at the moment and, believe me, I've tried them all and am always on the look-out for new teats on the market.

If you find milk is pouring out of the side of your baby's mouth while he is feeding then the flow may be too fast, the teat is not positioned correctly in your baby's mouth or he is not actively sucking and is potentially falling asleep. Equally if your baby is actively feeding but getting little milk reward then change to a faster flow or check the teat is not blocked. All the size one, slow flow teats have one small hole which can easily get blocked with milk. Clean the teats by turning them inside out or use a teat brush; rinse and squeeze water through so you can see the water spraying through the teat and that it is free-flowing. Changing to a size two teat should not be necessary in the first 2–3 months.

Sterilising

I believe we live in an over-sterile world and people are obsessed with antibacterial products. I personally don't use them unless I'm wiping down a baby's changing table or mat, but I do believe in keeping babies protected during the newborn stage and keeping good hygiene habits. Always wash your hands before feeding, dealing with baby bottles, after changing nappies or coming into your home from the outside world.

For the first 4–6 months, until you start weaning, you will need to sterilise all bottles, teats and breast pump attachments. For a single baby you can buy any option of steriliser. For twins or multiples I would buy a large electric steriliser like the Tommy Tippee Closer to Nature electric steam steriliser. Once the bottles have been sterilised, on emptying the steriliser, put the bottles and teats together so they are sealed – this will keep them sterilised until you use them. If you don't put them together once you have emptied the steriliser, the bottles will not remain sterile.

Sterilising bottles can stop once you start the weaning process. By then your baby will be putting everything in his mouth and be exposed to the wide range of bacteria needed to build a strong immune system.

Making up Feeds

There are four options for making up bottles in preparation for your baby's daily feeds. Always use fresh boiled water, not re-boiled, for making up your baby's bottles.

1. *Prepare all your bottles in advance.* Boil water and fill up the bottles. Leave to cool until it is warm or cool. Add the milk powder as advised on the formula box. Shake well and put the bottles in the fridge. Use within 24 hours and heat in a bottle warmer or a jug of boiling water. This option will take longer to heat the milk before a feed as you are heating it from cold.

2. *Make bottles as you go.* Boil water and fill up a bottle 15–20 minutes before a feed. Leave to cool down until it is the perfect temperature and then add milk powder just before the feed. Shake well to mix.

3. *Prepare bottles with water only.* Boil water and fill up the bottles. Leave sealed to cool for the day. 10–15 minutes before a feed add the milk powder to the cooled water, shake well and heat to the perfect temperature.

4. *My preferred way for easy instant milk …* Boil water and fill the bottles to just over halfway (if making up a 180ml (6oz) bottle, add 120ml (4oz) of boiling water). Seal the bottles and leave out (not in the fridge) until needed. Five to ten minutes before a feed, boil fresh water and add the remaining water needed, then add the milk powder and shake well. The temperature should be perfect and ready to go.

Heat your bottles using a bottle warmer or a jug of boiling water. Bear in mind that the milk will take longer to heat up from cold, so though the outside of the bottle may be hot, the milk inside could be cold, so test the temperature of the milk regularly. Please do not use a microwave to heat your baby's milk as it creates hot spots. As your feeds will be taking 45–60 minutes in the first two months, you will need to reheat the milk during the feed. Test the temperature of the milk, even if you reheat it during the feed. To do this, shake some milk on the inside of your wrist. If it stings the milk is too hot – it should feel warm or you should feel nothing. If the milk is too cool, it can make your baby gag and lose interest in feeding, not to mention being bad for his digestion and potentially giving him stomach ache. Warm milk is more digestible and more appealing for newborns.

It's worth noting that breast milk will heat up and cool down much quicker than formula. It will also flow faster through a teat being much thinner than formula.

How Long Will a Bottle-feed Take?

Bottle-feeding in the first few months of establishing feeding and increasing your baby's daily milk intake to the maximum intake of milk by Weeks 6–8 can take 45–60 minutes. Allowing an hour for feeds during the day will make sure your baby is full at each feed. The feeds should naturally speed up from eight weeks old as your baby's gut matures and he starts to become self-winding. This means he is able to take more milk between wind breaks and burps with ease.

During the establishing stage (the first 6–10 weeks of life) your newborn will need to be winded every 30ml (1oz). However, if he is excessively windy, he will need to be winded every 15–30ml (½–1oz). This amount of winding will make the feeds slower but will aid your baby's digestion and make for a more comfortable baby, which also allows a greater intake of milk having made more room for milk. Once your baby's gut matures (anytime from Week 8) he will be able to take 60ml (2oz) in one go before a wind break, increasing to 90ml (3oz) and so on until he needs winding only once or twice by the time he is around four months old. You will know when he is ready to do this as he will suddenly drink 60ml (2oz) of milk in the time he usually takes to drink 30ml (1oz). He may drink a greater volume of milk at the start of the feed and then drink less between winding breaks when he reaches the middle to the end of the feed, needing to be winded every 30ml (1oz).

Breaking to wind during the bottle-feed will make sure your baby doesn't take too much milk in one go, which can cause vomiting and trapped air which is unable to be relieved but has to pass through the intestines and out the other end which can cause pain. Taking too much milk too quickly is a bit like an adult drinking a glass of fizzy drink in one go – it causes indigestion and makes you feel like you are full. You could probably drink two or more glasses if you had sipped it at a slower rate over a longer period of time.

Feeding Position

Cradling your baby in your arms while feeding is lovely for cuddling and closeness once feeding is established. However, during the newborn stage, in a bid to keep your little one awake and actively feeding, try using a feeding pillow which helps to keep your baby supported and straight. As you can see below, this baby's head is in line with his back, not hanging forward or backwards, his bottom is supported and the teat is straight in his mouth with the bottle in line with his nose.

Poor feeding position can cause vomiting as, if the teat isn't straight, it will let in air. Don't be tempted to lift the teat up at the end of the feed so the teat is full of milk as this will let in air through the bottom of the teat as you lift the teat away from your baby's bottom lip. Feeding on a pillow leaves you with one hand free to stroke your baby's cheek or tickle his feet to help keep him awake and actively sucking during the feed. Your newborn can continuously drink until breaking to wind.

Slow and inactive feeding can result in poor milk intake. Your baby may become exhausted or even bored of feeding or start to comfort suck and fall asleep, taking not enough milk to see him through to the next feed, let alone through the night.

A newborn will generally not feed himself once he has taken the edge off his hunger or is dozing and falling asleep. Create the right feeding environment and position so you are able to have a free hand to prompt and keep your baby active while feeding. By 8–12 weeks old, your baby will be able to feed himself, become self-winding and able to stay awake during feeds.

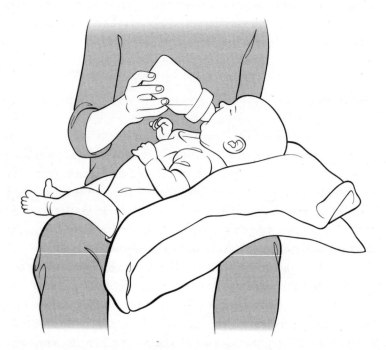

Ideal position for bottle-feeding

Milk Intake and Quantities

Formula-fed babies can often have longer intervals between feeds from the off, as formula milk is heavier, takes longer to digest and therefore sustains a baby for longer. Regardless of whether the bottle contains formula or expressed breast milk, you are aware of the quantity of milk your baby is taking and are able to gradually control the increase in his milk intake, which makes easy work of implementing a routine. Milk intake with breastfeeding is always a guesstimate. However, with a bottle you can accurately monitor the amount of milk your baby is taking, and this will vary, with some babies drinking much more milk than calculated for their age and weight. The general recommendation is 200ml (7oz) of milk for every kilogram of body weight per day, so if your baby weighs 3kg (6lb 9oz), he'll need about 600ml (21oz). These quantities are a guideline only and it's important to allow your newborn to increase his milk volume according to his appetite. Once you have increased your baby's milk intake, try not to backtrack on his daily quantities – if he needs less milk in a 24-hour period let the night feed be affected by this decrease.

Aim to feed your newborn every three hours for the first week of life only (see page 115), moving on to 3½–4-hourly feeding during the day with the 7pm to 7am Sleeping Baby Routine at Week 2 (see page 122). This aids digestion and encourages your baby's appetite for bigger feeds during the day, allowing enough time for awake/playtime and good-quality naps. Note that the time between feeds is measured from the beginning of one feed to the start of the next.

Your baby's daily milk intake will increase by an average of 15–30ml (½–1oz) per feed per week until he reaches the magic number of ounces he needs to sleep through the night. For some babies this will be 180–200ml (6–7oz) per feed, while for others it will be 240–290ml (8–10oz). The quantity needed to do this is personal to your baby and how fast and tall he is growing. Your baby has his fastest rate of growth in the first six weeks of life, so it is no wonder that babies can reach their maximum intake per feed by Weeks 6–8 and then plateau. Your baby will drink more during growth spurts, which generally occur at three weeks, six weeks and three months, though he may have 'mini growth spurts' each week.

The most important feed of the day is the post-bath, bedtime feed. This feed can be 60–90ml (2–3oz) larger than the morning feeds. This will enable longer periods of sleep during the night. Night feeds should never be more than 120ml (4oz), and the pre-bath bottle should be no more than 60ml (2oz) during the first 6–8 weeks. This is to encourage any increase of milk intake during the day and eventually phase out night feeds. The more milk you give overnight at any one feed, perhaps thinking to fill your baby up and for him to sleep longer, will have a knock-on effect and decrease the amount of milk he drinks during the day.

Always make bottles up to 30ml (1oz) more than your baby is usually taking to allow for an increase in appetite and to encourage him to take the majority of his milk during the day. Do this for every bottle during the day, but not for night feeds or the pre-bath bottle. Increasing your baby's milk intake during the day feeds in this way will decrease his appetite at night and eventually phase out night feeds. As you progress through the routine your baby will wake later through the night. When he starts waking past 3am start to reduce the amount of milk given:

- 11pm–3am: 120ml (4oz)
- 3am–4am: 90ml (3oz)
- 4am–5am: 60ml (2oz), keep your baby swaddled and no nappy change if possible
- 5am–6am: No feed zone. If after two minutes your baby hasn't settled back to sleep, keep him swaddled and cuddle, shush and hold him back to sleep (see Chapter Thirteen for more guidance). Ensure no lights are turned on and there is no other stimulation – be aware that monitor and camera light can be stimulating too

The pre-bath bottle

This can be increased to 90ml (3oz) after six weeks of age, but only if you have an extremely hungry baby who is taking 260ml (9oz) or more after the bath. Don't be tempted to give a larger feed for the pre-bath bottle as this is meant to be a snack only, which helps to make bath time calm, pleasant and fun. Too much milk before the bath can result in bloating, your baby being sick on the post-bath bottle and being disinterested in the biggest feed of the day, which is key to a peaceful night. Do take your time over this 60ml (2oz) pre-bath bottle and wind every 15ml (½oz) to slow it down otherwise it may be drunk so quickly your newborn's tummy won't realise it has been fed anything.

If your baby is still looking for food and seems dissatisfied with this restricted 60ml (2oz) feed, rest assured that he will get used to it as part of his routine. Distract him by taking him into the bathroom while you run the bath – the sound of running water will calm him – or walk around with him over your shoulder in the calming position (see page 206).

Wind

Bottle-fed babies tend to feed more efficiently as they don't have the flow issues that breastfed babies have. They often have much bigger burps and, if gulping, can get more trapped wind. A steady flow is therefore very important. Always make sure your baby is fully awake before winding him and wind him at least every 30ml (1oz) in the first six weeks. As your baby's tummy strengthens he will be able to manage more milk between burps and will start to self-wind at around

8–12 weeks. Babies who have excessive wind or are feeding quickly may need to be winded every 15ml (½oz). It may be worth switching to a lactose-free formula if you are noticing discomfort even when you are winding your baby properly and getting up lots of burps. Signs of excessive wind include: falling asleep and bloating soon after starting the feed, and vomiting. Formula-fed babies do not have the added benefit of probiotics through their mother's milk, so I advise adding a dose of infant probiotics to your baby's milk once a day to help strengthen his gut and boost immunity (see page 12).

Active Feeding

Bottle-fed babies tend to be more active when feeding than breastfed babies due to the constant flow of milk, but they can still start to doze off and lose focus – the sucking action alone is tiring in the first weeks of life and it's common for newborns to close their eyes while feeding. If they are still actively sucking, that is fine, but as they slow down or comfort suck they will drift off to sleep. It's important to prompt your baby to keep him actively sucking for the duration of the feed. Comfort sucking looks like a short up-and-down action, often with a shuddery jaw – nibble, nibble, pause, or long pause with the occasional suck. Active feeding looks like a wide circular motion with visible swallowing.

Allow one hour for feeding at each day feed as feeding too quickly and finishing a bottle of milk in less than 30 minutes can result in a milk slump, digestion issues, vomiting and an inability to wake your baby after feeds. Slow the feed down by winding your baby regularly, at 15–30ml (½–1oz) intervals, and use your spare hand to prompt him to keep your baby actively sucking. Don't allow dozing and comfort sucking which is bad for digestion and leads to ineffective feeding. Night feeds should be much quicker – around 20–30 minutes maximum for a nappy change, feed and winding. Your baby will be having less milk during the night feeds and will wake naturally so he should feed more efficiently.

Change your baby's nappy *after* the feed during the day as this will help him to wake and be ready for playtime, but change *before* feeds during the night to avoid stimulation and make it easier for your baby to settle back to bed.

I encourage a skin-on-skin nap once a day or at least once every two days, especially when bottle-feeding. Prop yourself in an elevated position with pillows under your arms, so you are unable to roll, and tuck yourself into bed with your baby naked (leave his nappy on!) lying on your chest and enjoy a snooze together. Get everything you need around you as you won't be able to move for the duration of the nap. Babies find it hard to wake from skin-on-skin naps so wake him up five minutes earlier, allowing 15–20 minutes to wake before feeding. (See page 197 for more on skin-on-skin naps.)

Chapter Eight

The Early Weeks

Week 1: Three-hourly Feeding

Your baby's routine in the first week will depend on how much she weighs and her appetite. Below is an example of a three-hourly routine. This routine starts at 7am, but you can choose the earlier start time of 6am to get an earlier night. This routine is *for the first week only*. Some premature babies may want to start on a four-hourly routine from birth giving them longer between feeds, and therefore more sleep, for maximum growth. Feeding three-hourly can be exhausting for a tiny baby and, as formula milk takes longer to digest, feeding four-hourly means they benefit from larger feeds less often.

If your baby is under 2.72kg (6lb) you may want to wake her for the first feed of the night between 10pm and 12am, until she reaches her birth weight, but ideally you should do this for no longer than a week as otherwise you will be setting your baby's body clock to wake and feed at around this time every evening.

The staggered bedtime feed is designed to be the biggest feed of the day and gives enough milk to sustain your baby until past 1am very quickly, leaving only one waking during the night. The nights should be baby-led: if your baby weighs over 2.72kg (6lb) and you are happy with her daily milk intake, let her wake naturally through the night. In my routine I encourage parents to wait two minutes when their baby wakes and cries to make sure she is truly ready for a feed (if she does not resettle back to sleep). See page 176 for more on my two-minute rule.

Week 1: Three-hourly Bottle-feeding Routine	
7am	60–120ml (2–4oz) bottle Total awake and playtime (including feed): 1–1½ hours
8/8.30am	Nap
10am	60–120ml (2–4oz) bottle Total awake and playtime (including feed): 1–1½ hours
11/11.30am	Nap
1pm	60–120ml (2–4oz) bottle Total awake and playtime (including feed): 1–1½ hours
2/2.30pm	Nap
4pm	60–120ml (2–4oz) bottle Total awake and playtime (including feed): 1–1½ hours
5/5.30pm	Nap
7pm	30–60ml (1–2oz) bottle maximum
7.15/7.30pm	Bath (34–35°C)
7.45/8pm	60–120ml (2–4oz) bottle
8.30/9pm	Bedtime (swaddled)
During the night	60–120ml (2–4oz) bottle maximum whenever your baby wakes Change your baby's nappy before the feed Swaddled for the last 30ml (1oz)

Notes on routine

- Milk intake and awake time will vary from baby to baby. Encourage a gradual increase of awake time until your baby reaches a full two hours at each day feed period, which should be easily obtained by around six weeks of age. Gradually increase your baby's daily milk intake until she reaches her own personal amount needed per feed to sleep through the night.

- Wake your baby 10–15 minutes before each day feed. Strip her down to a vest bodysuit to keep her cool for feeding. Use a feeding pillow to support your baby while feeding, which leaves one hand free to prompt her – by tickling her cheeks and feet – and encourage sucking.
- Allow an hour for feeds during the day and 30 minutes maximum during the night.
- Change your baby's nappy *after* feeding during the daytime to help wake her for playtime – time awake after feeds aids digestion. Using room temperature or cool water for her nappy change will encourage waking.
- Change your baby's nappy *before* feeding during the night-time. This avoids stimulation before settling.
- Swaddle your baby at night, but not during daytime naps unless she is very hard to settle or wakes frequently during naps. Tuck her in well in a cot, Moses basket or pram (see page 202 for more on this).
- Your baby's milk will need to be warmed and the temperature tested on the inside of your wrist. If it stings it is too hot; it should feel warm or you should feel nothing. If the milk is too cold it may give your baby stomach ache and be harder to digest, not to mention it will be less appealing to drink. Reheat during a feed as necessary.
- Wind your baby every 15–30ml (½–1oz) to relieve any discomfort from trapped air.

Weeks 2–3

Baby-led nights

Once your baby has regained her birth weight, is over 2.72kg (6lb) and is gaining weight, which should all happen at around Week 2, in contrast to your day routine you should let your baby wake of her own accord for feeds at night. This is where my technique differs from other baby experts who advise waking your baby on the dot for each feed day and night, or waking her for a 'dream feed' (a booster feed which is given before the parent would naturally go to bed). On my routine your nights are 'baby-led': if your baby is hungry, she will wake for a feed at night. By encouraging the majority of your baby's milk intake during the day, combined with the staggered feed and bottle at bedtime, there is no need to wake your baby for a dream feed. As your baby's day feeds and awake time increase over the weeks so will the length of time she sleeps at night, getting the much-needed rest to grow and thrive. As a result your baby will learn the difference between night and day very early on and night feeds will become efficient and short. You will also get the much-needed rest you need to recover and take care of your new baby.

Night feeds

Night waking and feeds should get gradually later with the increase in your baby's awake time and milk intake during the day. The later your baby wakes during the night, the less milk and less stimulation she should have during a night feed:

- 10pm–3am: 120ml (4oz), 20–30 minutes, swaddled for last 30ml (1oz)
- 3am–4am: 90ml (3oz), 20–30 minutes, swaddled for last 30ml (1oz)
- 4am–5am: 60–90ml (2–3oz), 10–15 minutes, keep swaddled for whole feed
- 5am–6am: No feed zone. Wait two minutes before reacting to waking and cuddle her back to sleep until 6am (see Chapter Four)

Keep your baby swaddled for any night feed after 4am, which keeps stimulation to a minimum and helps with settling back to sleep smoothly and quickly after the feed. There is no need to change your baby's nappy, unless it is dirty. By the time you reach this stage your newborn's body clock should have adjusted to only passing stools during the day.

If your baby has slept all the way through until 5am or 6am, she has slept the majority of the night so feeding at this time will be stimulating and she will most likely want a breakfast feed, not a snack, to get back to sleep. Feeding at this time will dramatically interfere with the 7am feed which can have a knock-on effect on your whole day routine. If your baby wakes at this time, keep her swaddled and cuddle her back to sleep by holding her on your chest firmly (cover up any naked skin which will only frustrate and not calm your baby – use a muslin or pop a top on), patting her back and bottom, and breathing deeply. This is a form of the 'shush and hold' technique (see page 205). As a very last resort, let your baby suck on your finger which will calm and soothe her. Stay in your baby's bedroom or go back to your bed in the dark. Start your day at 6am and switch your routine to the four-hourly 6am routine that day. This is the only time of day I would advise letting your baby suck your finger or cuddling your baby back to sleep as I don't believe in babies sucking for comfort. It creates wind and has a negative effect on the morning feed.

Keep all lights as low as possible during night feeds and avoid talking to your baby or giving her any kind of stimulation so that she can settle more easily back to sleep. Feed your baby, wind her and put her straight back to bed – this will help to teach her the difference between night and day.

Try not to react straight away if you hear your baby crying. Use the two-minute rule to see if she is truly ready to be fed or whether she settles back to sleep. The two-minute rule should be used night and day for sleep, naps and playtime. During the night some babies grizzle, stretch and grunt for a while before waking properly, but please let your baby grizzle undisturbed. The chances are that she is still in 'sleep mode' with her eyes closed. If you rush in to feed your baby whenever you hear a cry or grizzle, you are not allowing her a chance to resettle. You may be starting a feed she is not ready for, only for her to wake again a few hours later when she is actually ready for milk. At night, babies go through lots of lighter periods of sleep and during those light periods they can twitch, turn, grizzle, and even cry a bit, but if left for two minutes they will often go back to sleep if swaddled and tucked in. This encourages self-settling.

Top tips for night feeding

- Keep your baby's room dark, using blackout blinds in the summer, and with no night light. Keep the camera monitor light covered as it will shine straight on to your baby's face. Once she has reached six weeks and wakes in the night, any light, albeit dim lighting, will stimulate her. Night lights can be used, if at all, much later on, at around six months plus.
- Keep night feeds in the same room as your baby sleeps in. Moving rooms, turning lights on and walking around are stimulating and will encourage waking. Practise short, dark, quiet feeds with no talking, phones or TV.
- Swaddle your baby at night until she is sleeping through the night for at least two weeks. If she wakes and the swaddle is loose or her arms have come out, this may be the only reason for waking and she will not be able to resettle with her arms waving around. Re-swaddle her, give her a cuddle and then pop her back to bed. Regardless of the reason for waking, a newborn will immediately think 'milk', so you may need to feed her if re-swaddling and resettling doesn't work. The swaddle technique is key to your baby settling! Tuck her into bed with no loose blankets. Babies feel secure, cuddled and sleep better if they are wrapped and firmly tucked in.

This also helps to stop her waking due to the startle reflex. (See pages 198 and 202 for more advice on swaddling and tucking in.)

- Change your baby's nappy *before* night feeds. Changing her nappy after a feed will again stimulate her and encourage waking, making it more difficult for her to settle back to sleep.
- Night feeds should take no longer than 30 minutes. The idea is to change your baby, feed her and then put her back to bed quickly. The length and quantity of feeds should decrease the later your baby wakes (see page 64). This is to help phase out night feeds and to not interfere with the morning feed at 7am. The maximum for any one night feed is capped at 120ml (4oz) from a bottle.
- Swaddle your baby for the last five minutes of the night feed and let her drift to sleep, winding her over your shoulder and then promptly putting her back to bed.

Room temperature

It's important to ensure that your baby does not overheat or get too cold. If a baby is cold she will wake; if she is too hot overheating becomes more of a danger. Everyone thinks that it's necessary to keep a baby warm with lots of layers, even putting on hats and mittens indoors, because babies are unable to regulate their own temperature. However, this is usually for the first few weeks of life until they start gaining weight and body fat. Even so, babies release heat through their skin so it's important to keep the room temperature above 18°C degrees at all times and not use hats indoors.

The ideal sleeping environment is a room temperature of 18–21°C with your baby dressed in a vest bodysuit, a Babygro or sleepsuit, a swaddle, roll pillows (if using) and one thick, stretchy blanket or two thinner blankets to tuck her in (see Chapter Thirteen for more on swaddling, sleep positions and tucking in). If in the summer months the temperature goes up, reduce the layers by removing the sleepsuit/Babygro first and use a thinner blanket to tuck your baby in. You should always keep the swaddle and a thin blanket, or even a large muslin, to tuck her in. If the room temperature reaches over 24°C look to cool it down by letting air in or using a fan, with the air flow not directly on your baby.

The ideal feeding/awake time temperature is 19–20°C. This is a little warmer than the sleeping temperature because I advise babies to be fed in a vest bodysuit, which means their arms and legs are exposed, but the room should be no hotter than 20°C as babies heat up while they are feeding and digesting.

Below are two examples of the 7pm to 7am Sleeping Baby Routine for bottle-fed babies. The first has flexible feed timings, while the second is a non-flexible four-hourly feeding routine. The milk quantity is based on a two-week-old baby weighing 2.72–4.08kg (6–9lb).

Weeks 2–3: 3½–4-hourly Bottle-feeding Routine	
7am	120–180ml (4–6oz) bottle Total awake and playtime (including feed): 1½–2 hours
8.30/9am	Nap
10.30/11am	120–180ml (4–6oz) bottle Total awake and playtime (including feed): 1½–2 hours
12/1pm	Nap
2.30pm	120–180ml (4–6oz) bottle Total awake and playtime (including feed): 1½–2 hours

4/4.30pm	Nap
6pm	60ml (2oz) bottle
6.30pm	Bath (34–35°C)
6.45pm	120–180ml (4–6oz) bottle
7.15/8pm	Bedtime (swaddled)
During the night	90–120ml (3–4oz) bottle maximum whenever your baby wakes Wind every 30ml (1oz) Change your baby's nappy before the feed Swaddled for the last 30ml (1oz)

Weeks 2–3: Four-hourly Bottle-feeding Routine

6am	120–180ml (4–6oz) bottle Total awake and playtime (including feed): 1½–2 hours
7.30/8am	Nap
10am	120–180ml (4–6oz) bottle Total awake and playtime (including feed): 1½–2 hours
11.30/12pm	Nap
2pm	90–150ml (3–5oz) bottle Total awake and playtime (including feed): 1½–2 hours
3.30/4pm	Nap
6pm	60ml (2oz) maximum
6.30pm	Bath (34–35°C)
6.45pm	120–180ml (4–6oz) bottle
7.30pm	Bedtime (swaddled)
During the night	90–120ml (3–4oz) bottle maximum whenever your baby wakes Wind every 30ml (1oz) Change your baby's nappy before the feed Swaddled for the last 30ml (1oz)

Notes on routine

- Milk intake and awake time will vary from baby to baby. Encourage a gradual increase of awake time until your baby reaches a full two hours at each day feed period, which should be easily obtained by around six weeks of age. Gradually increase your baby's daily milk intake until she reaches her own personal amount needed per feed to sleep through the night.
- Wake your baby 10–15 minutes before each day feed. This ensures she is fully awake, ready to eat and focused, which encourages active feeding.
- Gradually increase your baby's awake time to two hours at each feed period throughout the coming week. The time is taken from the start of the feed, not the 10–15 minute waking up period before the feed.
- Allow an hour maximum for day feeds, which includes winding. This will of course speed up as your baby grows and her gut strengthens but, until she is sleeping through the night, make use of that hour to make sure she is full and winded well.
- Do not wake your baby for night feeds after her bedtime bottle, but let her wake naturally for a feed. Night feeds should be at least four hours apart.
- Change your baby's nappy *after* feeding during the daytime, to help wake her for playtime.
- Change your baby's nappy *before* feeding during the night. If she is waking only once at night, try to avoid changing her nappy unless it is dirty. Try using a larger size nappy for nights to accommodate a full night's sleep without changing. Make sure the nappy is fitted securely around the legs to prevent any leaks. If your baby is waking more than once, change her nappy at the first waking only.
- Swaddle your baby when you put her to bed at night, but not during daytime naps unless she is hard to settle or wakes often during naps.

- Wind your baby well, every 30ml (1oz) and maybe every 15ml (½oz) as she reaches the end of the bottle, making sure she is wide awake while winding. You will also need to check for burps and wind during playtime while she is digesting the feed. Remember: digestion creates wind (see page 7).

Chapter Nine

Week 4 Onwards

The bottle-feeding routine remains the same now until your baby is weaned at 4–6 months. The only changes will be fluctuations of milk intake and less sleep during the day. Each week the quantity of milk intake is increased until your baby has reached the quantity he personally needs to sleep through the night, which I have found, over the last 20 years, to be anywhere between 200ml (7oz) and 260ml (9oz) per feed. The increase is gradual and only by 15–30ml (½–1oz) per feed per week. By Week 2 you will know where your baby's appetite sits and be feeding him a consistent amount at each feed, which is usually around 120ml (4oz) per feed. This is the starting point to start gradually increasing his milk intake. The following routine gradually increases your baby's awake time at each feed period until you reach two hours at each feed and, with some wakeful babies, 2¼ hours.

I find it helps to focus on a baby's awake time rather than the number of hours he has slept during the day. A baby on my routine who sleeps solidly at night will not need as much sleep during the day as a baby who wakes 1–4 times a night. Often day naps become unsettled the longer and deeper the sleep is at night. The afternoon nap is the first to become unsettled as early as 4–6 weeks of age and some babies naturally drop it from Week 8 or find it hard to sleep at this period of the day. When this starts to happen adjust the routine, leaving a shorter gap between the afternoon feed and pre-bath feed of 3–3½ hours. This gives a longer awake time and a shorter nap: doing the afternoon feed at 3pm gives only a 45-minute window for your baby to sleep. Make the afternoon feed 30ml (1oz) less than the morning feeds. This will help build a bigger appetite for the evening feed which will eventually be 30–60ml (1–2oz) more than the morning feed, becoming the largest feed of the day and setting your baby up for a full night's sleep.

Be flexible

The 7pm to 7am Sleeping Baby Routine allows your routine to be flexible but also, by ending each day at the same time, encourages consistency which is important in enabling your baby to recognise that bedtime is coming, which helps to set his body clock to sleep well. Below are some alternative routine feed timings which all end with the same bedtime:

- 6am, 10am, 2pm, 6pm pre-bath feed, 6.30pm bath, 6.45pm feed, 7.30pm bed
- 6.30am, 10/10.30am, 2/2.30pm, 6pm pre-bath feed, 6.30pm bath, 6.45pm feed, 7.30pm bed
- 7am, 10.30/11am, 2.30pm, 6pm pre-bath feed, 6.30pm bath, 6.45pm feed, 7.30pm bed
- 7am, 11am, 2.30/3pm, 6pm pre-bath feed, 6.30pm bath, 6.45pm feed, 7.30pm bed
- 7.30am, 11/11.30am, 3pm, 6pm pre-bath feed, 6.30pm bath, 6.45pm feed, 7.30pm bed

The amount of milk intake will vary with some babies drinking much more milk than calculated for their age and weight. The general rule is 200ml (7oz) of milk per kilogram of body weight, but these quantities are a guideline so allow your baby to increase his milk volume according to his appetite. If you give less milk than needed per feed during the day he will naturally wake to take it at night, so be consistent with day quantities and increase until night feeds are phased out.

Keep a baby routine diary

The easiest way is to buy a diary that has one day per page. This helps you to see the pattern that is developing and work out your routine for each day.

Playtime and stimulation

By now you should really be enjoying playtime with your baby and starting to get a few smiles. Your baby may start to track and follow so using a cot mobile for awake time and toys dangling from the arches of a play mat may start to hold interest, but most babies are still more interested in black-and-white images and their parents' faces. A baby's attention span shortens as the weeks go by with the ability to see at a distance and follow movement, and static black-and-white toys will no longer offer the same entertainment by Weeks 6–8. Your baby may decide that the best place to be is with you, being carried around and complaining about being put down to play. It is important, however, that he still has some time playing on his own and is not being picked up and put down every few minutes when he grizzles. It will only make for a more demanding and insecure baby who is less able to play by himself. Whenever your baby cries to be picked up, use your voice to soothe him, rotate his toys, try tummy time or move him to a different area of the house – perhaps in his chair where he can watch you. Simply holding your baby's feet can give him security of your touch and will often calm and distract. Toys with squeaky and rustle sounds, such as the Lamaze Jacques the Peacock, are also a big favourite at this time.

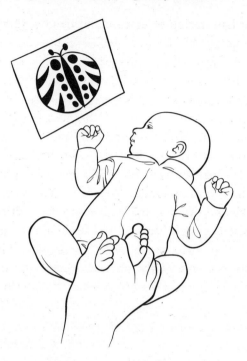

Holding feet to reassure and calm baby during playtime

The first half of playtime is the best time for self-play, so put your baby down to play on a play mat while you look after yourself. Ensure you don't give your baby tummy time sooner than 30 minutes after a feed, as you need to allow time for digestion. The end of the playtime, as your baby starts to get tired and grumpy and needs distracting, can be reserved for one-on-one chat time with you. Finally enjoy a cuddle before his nap. Remember to check for wind during your baby's playtime. Wind is formed while digesting milk and can be the cause of grizzles or falling asleep during playtime. Most newborns therefore need to burp a few times before going down for a nap.

Once your baby is sleeping through the night and has reached his maximum milk intake, you will need to be consistent with your routine to maintain results. Your routine at 6–8 weeks should now require less effort as feeds speed up as your baby's gut has started to mature and he now starts to become self-winding, is able to stay awake with ease, settles himself for naps and by Weeks 8–10 starts being able to stay awake in motion, which takes all restrictions out of your previous daily routine. From Weeks 10–12 your baby's rate of growth will have started to slow a little and his appetite will plateau. The longer your baby sleeps through the night the more flexible feeds become as his appetite will go up and down slightly by 30–60ml (1–2oz) per feed. Try and keep the bedtime bottle consistent. Allow your routine to become much more flexible with milk intake and timings, but do keep to the bedtime routine to keep consistency with bedtime and sleeping through the night.

Below is an example of the 7pm to 7am Sleeping Baby Routine for bottle-fed babies at 6–8 weeks. The milk quantity is based on a baby weighing 4.08–4.98kg/9–11lb.

Week 4 Onwards: The 7pm to 7am Sleeping Baby Routine	
7am	180–240ml (6–8oz) bottle Total awake and playtime (including feed): 2–2¼ hours
9/9.15am	Nap
10.30/11am	180–240ml (6–8oz) bottle Total awake and playtime (including feed): 2–2¼ hours
12.30/1.15pm	Nap
2.30pm	180–200ml (6–7oz) bottle Total awake and playtime (including feed): 2–2¼ hours
4.30/4.45pm	Nap
6pm	60ml (2oz) bottle
6.30pm	Bath (34–35°C)
6.45pm	180–240ml (6–8oz) bottle
7.15/8pm	Bedtime (swaddled)

During the night	11pm–3am: 90–120ml (3–4oz) maximum
	3am–4am: 90ml (3oz) maximum
	4am–5am: 60–90ml (2–3oz), keep baby swaddled
	5am–6am: No feed zone
	Wind every 30ml (1oz)

Notes on routine

- Milk intake and awake time will vary from baby to baby. Encourage a gradual increase of awake time until your baby reaches a full two hours at each day feed period, which should be easily obtained by around six weeks of age. Gradually increase your baby's daily milk intake until he reaches his own personal amount needed per feed to sleep through the night.
- If your baby is still waking in the night at this stage try reducing his milk intake at the night feeds.
- If he is waking at the same time during the night out of habit, try resettling instead of automatically feeding after leaving for the two-minute rule.
- By now your baby should be able to stay awake for two hours at each feed period if you have started my routine from the off. If your baby is unsettled during naps, increase this to 2¼ hours to help combat this. He may also need much less sleep during the day if he is solidly sleeping through the night. This isn't a problem if he is happy to wait for feeds so you can keep to similar timings.

Implementing a Routine at a Later Stage

Many of you will be reading this book because you have run into problems with on-demand feeding and now want to try to encourage your baby into a routine. The flexibility of my routine makes this quite simple. If your baby is snacking and taking small quantities of milk frequently, he will need to increase his milk intake gradually. The greater your baby's appetite and the greater his milk intake, the longer the milk intake will sustain him between feeds. If you are bottle-feeding and formula feeding go straight to the 7pm–7am routine if you are past the three-week mark, then increase all day feeds by 30ml (1oz) at a time. It may take a while for your baby to get used to taking more milk at each feed if he is currently used to snacking. If he is sleeping a great deal in the day, wake him for feeds and try to keep him awake afterwards for as long as you can, aiming for two hours at each feed period and building the routine gradually. Do not let him go more than four hours between feeds during the day. Conversely, at night he should not be fed more often than four-hourly. Stagger the bedtime feed, splitting it with a bath as suggested, to increase his milk intake before bed. The case study on page 84 shows how quickly you can turn things round from chaos to calm.

Months 4–6 Onwards

My routine will take you up to the weaning stage. The only differences with the routine between the newborn stage and the now established baby stage are:

1. *The length of sleep needed during the day is reduced.* Your baby may have already dropped his afternoon nap or be having a very short one. The length of sleep a baby needs during the day varies from baby to baby, but the general focus should be on a longer lunchtime nap of 1½–2 hours. Keeping this nap in your baby's cot as much as possible, and therefore providing the right sleeping environment, will help keep this nap solid. This lunchtime nap will stay part of your child's routine until he is around three years old. If for any reason your baby's lunchtime nap is unsettled, extend his morning awake time to 2½–3 hours

and reduce his morning nap to increase the length of sleep he has over the middle of the day, which in turn will help to reduce and phase out the afternoon nap. The morning nap should be 30–60 minutes long.

Once your baby has dropped his afternoon nap, you might find that you need to bring the pre-bath feed earlier to 5.30pm, but still keep to the bath time of 6.30pm. The post-bath bottle should now be super-efficient and your baby should be going to bed nearer to 7pm.

2. *Sleep position.* Your baby will now be sleeping in a cot and possibly moving around and sleeping in a sleeping bag. Keep your baby tucked in for as long as he is not moving. Babies who move around and roll in their cot too early often get stuck in positions and then wake and cry out for help to move them back.

3. *Your routine is now much more flexible* and you are able to feed your baby while out and about. Your baby can now stay awake in motion so you are no longer restricted to only going out at nap times, and his awake and playtimes can often be on the move or during activities such as meeting friends or baby groups.

4. *Feed times and quantities can be flexible* as your baby's appetite goes up and down, but don't change your baby's bath and bottle times as it is important to be consistent with bedtime. This part of the routine will not change until your baby is a child and his bedtime bottle is replaced with story time. When bottle-feeding, the amount of milk taken between burps increases to 60–90ml (2–3oz), which speeds up the length of feeding time. If your baby is not yet sleeping through the night, still allow an hour for each day feed.

Weaning

Though the blanket advice from the Department of Health is to wean your baby at six months (26 weeks) of age, I do things a little differently and, if necessary, wean babies on to solid food ever so slowly from four months. Research evidence has proven that babies are digestively ready to be weaned on to solid food between four and six months, but, for some reason, the government advice has been set at six months. Waiting until six months with a baby who is ready to be weaned from four months will cause night waking, disruptive days and frustration, which may be mistaken for teething which occurs at around the same time. Starting solids as soon as you see the signs that your baby is ready (see below) means that you are able to take a slower approach to introducing solid food, which is, of course, better for your baby's digestion.

As babies get older, they have much more of an opinion on everything, including what goes into their mouths. There is certainly a difference between a baby of four months and a baby of six months in this respect. Starting weaning at six months often means it can be a stressful process as it's a rush to get your baby fully weaned as quickly as possible. A baby who is actually ready for food from four months can spend two weeks simply introducing a few spoons at one meal a day, and this gives you time to build the quantities. For those of you with babies who are not ready to wean until 5–6 months, enjoy the ease of milk feeding as it all gets a bit messy from here on in!

Below are signs to look out for when deciding if your baby is ready to be weaned:

- *Your baby starts waking at night having slept through for the last month or so.* He wakes due to hunger but is not interested in upping his milk intake during the day. At around four months some babies can lose interest in their milk. Night waking is believed to be the result of a growth spurt, but in my experience a growth spurt often means a baby is more hungry or sleeps more, so if your baby is waking having slept through for months, it makes sense that his food intake should be the first thing to address. Some mothers who are breastfeeding look to introduce formula as a stopgap to satisfy their baby until they are ready to start weaning.

- *Your baby is very interested in watching you eat* and often dribbles while watching you and will look like he is chewing. This is not the same as your baby chewing on his hands, as all babies do this as soon as they are able to and while teething.
- *Your baby can hold his own head up and sit when supported.*
- *Your baby dramatically goes off his milk or is no longer satisfied with his milk intake during the day.* Yes, milk has more calories than puréed carrot but it is liquid and won't sustain your baby as long as solid food will. It takes weeks to build the amount of solid food a baby takes, so weaning is initially a supplement to your baby's milk.
- *Your baby can swallow.* Babies who aren't yet ready to be weaned will still have the tongue thrust reflex, which pushes food out of their mouths before swallowing.

Please talk to your health visitor or GP for advice if you feel your baby is ready to be introduced to solid food before six months.

PART THREE

Twins

Chapter Ten

Twins Routine

Twins are my thing! I started this journey specialising in baby sleep routines 20 years ago with newborn twins and, having mostly twins in my care for the first five years, I fast became a specialist in twin routines. Double trouble? No, double the joy! Of course, you do need to plan ahead, be organised and prepared, but with both babies on the same routine, doing everything together at the same time, it is not too different from having one baby; it's just that everything takes half an hour longer.

Twins can be easier to establish on a routine as they are usually born on the small side so tend to need more sleeping time to grow, which means they will naturally sleep longer at night. Try to take advantage of this: if your babies are under 2.72kg (6lb), then wake them for a night feed, but allow longer stretches of sleep at night, between four and six hours, so that you are teaching them the difference between night and day straight away. Vary the time you wake them so you don't set their body clocks to naturally wake at a certain time during the night. Once they are over 2.72kg (6lb), wake them only once in the night between 11pm and 2am until they are both gaining weight and are back to their birth weights; only then can you let them wake naturally for the night feed.

Despite being small and often premature, you can introduce a routine for twins from birth. Even premature babies, weighing only around 1.8kg (4lb), are put on to a three- to four-hourly feeding routine in hospital. If your babies are over

2.72kg (6lb) and putting on weight nicely, there is no reason why you cannot start my 7pm to 7am Sleeping Baby Routine with baby-led nights. If you do not feel comfortable with this and wish to wake your twins for a night feed in the first two weeks then, again, vary the waking time so as not to set a pattern of waking during the night.

The reason a routine for twins is a mixed feeding routine is that, when breastfeeding, you will eventually need 1½–2 'breasts-full' per feed – a bit tricky when you only have the two breasts! Many mothers struggle to produce enough milk for one baby let alone two and, although it is possible to feed twins exclusively on the breast for a while, this may mean feeding every 2–3 hours day and night. Topping up with expressed breast milk or formula gives you the guarantee your babies are full at each feed, will make lighter work of implementing a routine and ensure your babies sleep at night.

Tandem feeding (page 143) is key to the success of your routine, keeping your babies in sync and sleeping well at night. Start this as early on as you can. As your babies grow they will get heavier and move around so it is best to get used to tandem feeding while they are small and not yet on the move.

Adapting the Routines for Twins

The twins' routines are exactly the same in principle as a single baby routine, with the difference being your breastfeed is up to 30 minutes (rather than an hour) as it will take no longer than 30 minutes to drain one breast. Follow either the mixed feeding routine (page 93), also reading Chapter Two (page 27), or the bottle-feeding routine (see Part Two, page 99). Wake both babies up at the same time for feeds, put them down for their naps at the same time and do everything together as much as possible. The nights may be a bit tricky for a while, as twins often appear to take it in turns to wake for feeds. You may find that one twin will be the first to wake for a week, then the other will take over for a while. Regardless of which twin wakes in the night for feeds, get them both up to feed at the same time or you will exhaust yourself being awake all night, feeding them one at a time.

As with all my routines, the aim is to encourage your babies to sleep through the night and, with twins, it's even more important not to 'backtrack' once you start to make progress. By this I mean that once the twins have started to fall into a pattern of waking at, say, 1am for a week, and then they start randomly waking earlier one night, try not to feed them but instead resettle them until after their usual waking time. The next day make sure the early waking twin has increased her milk intake and had enough awake time at each feed period. Your twins will most likely have growth spurts at different stages so their ability to stay awake for the duration of play-time and their appetites may differ. Work out what they are capable of individually in terms of milk intake and awake time, then build on and increase this until they can both stay awake for the full two-hour period. Also increase their milk intake during the day until they are sleeping through the night.

Once your babies are sleeping through the night and they have reached their maximum milk intake, you will need to be consistent with your routine to maintain results. By Week 8 your routine should now require less effort as feeds speed up as your babies' guts start to mature and they now start to become self-winding, are able to stay awake with ease, settle themselves for naps and by Weeks 10–12 start to stay awake in motion, which takes all restrictions out of your previous daily routine. From Weeks 10–12 your babies' rate of growth will have started to slow a little and their appetites will plateau. The longer your babies sleep through the night the more flexible feeds become as their appetites will go up and down slightly. So, once they are established and coming out of the newborn stage, allow your routine to become more flexible with milk intake and timings, but do keep to the bedtime routine to keep consistency with bedtime and sleeping through the night.

Dummies

Although I do not recommend using dummies as they teach the wrong association with sucking, cause wind and digestive discomfort, and create a bad habit, I occasionally use them with twins as a temporary measure and only when they are both close to sleeping through the night; that is, when one twin is sleeping through and the other is still waking or they take it in turns to sleep through. For example, I would use a dummy if both babies were waking at 5am but their feed was not due until 6am, they had been waking at the same time for four or five nights and a habit of waking had been formed. This usually happens at around Weeks 6–8. Only use the dummy for a maximum of one week otherwise you will be stuck with it and then have the problem of your babies waking due to the dummy falling out, which could lead to you being awake in the night more often than ever before. The dummy trick will either work or it won't, so, either way, stop using it. If it doesn't work with settling or does work and waking issues are resolved, then throw it away! If you have a dummy around the house and have two whingeing babies at any point you may be tempted to use it which can create lots of problems within the routine. Only use the dummy when you have a consistent pattern – it should be the last resort in sleep training.

The two-minute rule

During the small wee hours of the night, a baby crying for two minutes can feel like 10 minutes because it is the only thing you can hear. As with a single baby, you should not jump to your babies' every cry. This self-control can be harder with twins as you may worry that one crying baby will wake the other. I find that it's not the crying that wakes the other twin but when they stop crying. You need to leave any crying for two minutes before reacting to see if your baby settles. Your twins may take it in turns to cry out, which can sound like they are awake for longer than they actually are when, in fact, they have only cried for a minute or so each and have resettled. You should be able to recognise the difference between each baby's cry quite early on.

Tandem Feeding

Tandem feeding allows you to feed both babies at the same time so they keep to the same schedule, which allows you to have the same amount of downtime as parents of a single baby. The routine is exactly the same as for a single baby, but may take a little longer when feeding and winding two babies, meaning day feeds – handling two babies to wind and feed – can take an extra 15 minutes at each feed.

When tandem feeding, each twin will have a whole breast each. Swap your starting breast for each baby at each feed, and then top up with expressed milk or formula until both babies are full. You should quickly get into a pattern of their milk intake. If your milk supply increases you will see a very slow increase in the milk your babies are taking at the top-up feed. If this doesn't happen, or when your supply stops increasing, increase their top-up bottles by 30ml (1oz) per feed per week until they are sleeping through the night.

If you are using both expressed milk and formula for top-ups, use the expressed milk during the night firstly, then for the afternoon feed. Breast milk digests quicker and is a lighter feed than formula, and the aim is to encourage lighter feeds during the night and in the afternoon in order to build an appetite for the biggest feed of the day before bed. Formula should be given at the post-bath bedtime bottle as it is heavier and will sustain your babies for longer. It's commonly thought that giving heavier feeds during the night will help your babies sleep longer at night, but this is simply not the case long-term. Instead, what this will do is encourage night waking for a big feed. Make sure you cap the night feeds at 120ml (4oz) maximum at any one feed or 20–30 minutes in total if you are breastfeeding. If you are finding you don't have enough milk for a breastfeed alone, then give a 15–20-minute breastfeed and top up with a maximum of 30–60ml (1–2oz) to help settle your babies. The later they wake through the night, the more of a milk build-up you have and the more likely one breast will satisfy. If you have two night feeds, one could be a breastfeed and the other a 120ml (4oz) maximum bottle of expressed breast milk.

Breastfeeding, bottle-feeding and expressing with two babies is a lot of work for a mother so the second express (mid-morning) is optional. It's still important to understand your milk supply so expressing after the morning feeds and in the evening will help you get to know your breasts, your milk flow and supply, while making sure your supply is tip-top. Expressing will also allow you a comfortable night as your babies sleep later through the night.

If you want to encourage a good milk supply and give your babies as much breast milk as possible, use the breast-feeding option during the night or for at least one of the night feeds if you have two night feeds. The bottle-feeding option for the nights is easier, but, as mentioned above, use breast milk here where possible to encourage lighter feeds during the night.

For tandem feeding you will need a sofa to feed your babies; one in the nursery for night feeds will make your life much easier. Tandem breastfeeding pillows only work if you have smaller, high breasts, but they are great if you can use them. Alternatively, two large, square pillows work well. Make sure the square pillows are firm and keep your babies raised, not sunken into the pillow. You may need a smaller pillow for support underneath. The pillows are slightly supported by your legs so your babies' heads are higher than their bottoms either side of you.

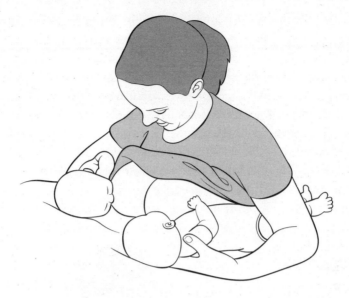

Ideal position for tandem breastfeeding

Tandem feeding allows you to keep your babies on track and in sync with each other routine-wise. In the early weeks babies tend not to move, so tandem feeding is easy in that respect, but it means you don't have the spare hand to prompt and keep your babies actively sucking. If you are bottle-feeding, hold the bottles lower down the bottle, closer to the teat so you can use your fingers to stroke their cheeks for encouragement. When one twin becomes inactive, take the bottle out and use your feeding hand to tickle her awake if the other twin is still actively drinking. This means you are not leaving the inactive twin to drift off to sleep, which will have an impact on playtime and naps. Leaving one twin sleeping while you are feeding the other encourages catnapping. Once the active twin starts to slow down, break them both for a wind break to help regain focus and encourage active feeding.

Once your babies start to move, with their arms and legs kicking and waving around out of control, their heads are able to turn away from the bottle and their stomach muscles start developing, you may be able to start the feed by tandem feeding for the first 90–150ml (3–5oz) and then need to feed one baby at a time, swapping them every 30–60ml (1–2oz). They will become increasingly harder to tandem feed as they get older. Moving forward with the bottle you can move to baby chairs to feed, sitting yourself between the two. Another option is to feed separately giving the most enthusiastic twin 30–60ml (1–2oz) to take the edge off her hunger and then swapping babies every 30–60ml (1–2oz). Tandem feeding where possible is your best option for keeping your babies on track for a successful routine.

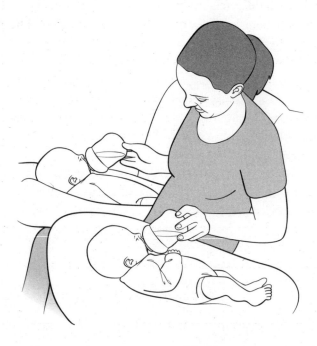

Ideal position for tandem bottle-feeding

Make up the bottles for top-ups before you start the breastfeed so they are ready to go. The milk will need to be warmed and the temperature tested on the inside of your wrist. If it stings it is too hot; it should feel warm or you should feel nothing. If the milk is too cold it can give your baby a stomach ache and be harder to digest, not to mention it is less appealing to drink. Leave both bottles in hot water, or a controlled temperature bottle warmer, to keep them at the perfect temperature for a quick change from breast to bottle. Wind your babies after every 5–10 minutes on the breast or every 15–30ml (½–1oz) on the bottle.

Your twin babies may vary dramatically in size but this doesn't mean that the smaller twin will feed less. More often than not the smaller twin will have a bigger appetite in a race to catch up with her sibling. Your baby's size doesn't always determine the amount of milk you should give so try and keep both babies feeding around the same quantity of milk which will help keep them on the same routine. The intake only usually differs by 30ml (1oz) between babies. Wake them both at the same time, keep them awake for the same amount of time and put them to bed at the same time. Some days this might be tricky, much like keeping a single baby awake and on a routine, and they may have growth spurts at slightly different stages, but aim to encourage them both to feed, wind and have some awake time at each feed period.

Weeks 3–5: Mixed Feeding Routine for Twins	
7am	Tandem breastfeed for 25–30 minutes + 30–90ml (1–3oz) formula
8/8.15am	Express Total awake and playtime (including feed): 2 hours
9am	Nap
10.30/11am	Tandem breastfeed for 25–30 minutes + 60–120ml (2–4oz) expressed breast milk/ formula
11.30am/12.15pm	Express Total awake and playtime (including feed): 1½–2 hours

1/2.15pm	Nap
2.30pm	Tandem breastfeed for 20–30 minutes + 90–120ml (3–4oz) expressed breast milk/ formula Total awake and playtime (including feed): 1½–2 hours
4/4.30pm	Nap
6pm	Tandem breastfeed for 20–30 minutes
6.30pm	Bath (34–35°C)
6.45pm	120–180ml (4–6oz) formula
7.15/8pm	Bedtime (swaddled)
9/9.30pm	Express
During the night	11pm–3am: 90–120ml (3–4oz) bottle maximum or breastfeed for 30 minutes 3am–4am: 90ml (3oz) maximum or breastfeed for 20 minutes 4am–5am: 60–90ml (2–3oz) bottle maximum or breastfeed for 10–15 minutes, keep babies swaddled 5am–6am: No feed zone Wind every 30ml (1oz) or 5 minutes on the breast

Notes on routine

- Milk intake and awake time will vary from baby to baby. Encourage a gradual increase of awake time until your babies reach a full two hours at each day feed period, which should be easily obtained by around six weeks of age. Gradually increase your babies' daily milk intake until they reach their own personal amount needed per feed to sleep through the night.
- Getting organised and using your time efficiently will result in you being able to rest and get out and about. Before waking your babies 10–15 minutes before each

feed, get one step ahead and make yourself a drink and a snack or prepare lunch to have while the babies are playing happily after their feed.

- Wake up in the morning 20 minutes before waking them for the day to have a shower and a cuppa. Have breakfast and lunch while the babies are playing before they nap, which will allow you the time to go out, rest or have skin-on-skin nap time with one of your babies.

Jack and Samuel's story

I arrived in the beautiful Peak District to help troubleshoot unsettled twin boys, Jack and Samuel, aged nine weeks old. The twins were already on a routine of structured feeding, being breastfed every three hours, but separately, and being topped up with a bottle of formula if and when they were not settling. They were not sleeping or settling well, they grunted, grizzled and were constantly passing wind, which gives the indication they were being fed too frequently, were not being winded frequently or may be sensitive to Mum's diet. It was clear that wind and digestion were at least some of the reasons for their unsettled daytime naps – they were uncomfortable and needed to be winded more frequently during feeds. The boys were also waking three times a night. As soon as they cried out during the night, Mum was rushing in to feed, cuddle or rock them back to sleep, in the hope she could settle the crying twin quickly so he wouldn't wake his brother. As a result the boys had not learned how to settle themselves. The twins were also being put to bed with their arms out and not tucked into their cot.

After assessing the situation for a few hours, we started putting my plan into action:

- Changing Mum's diet while breastfeeding: this would make a huge difference to the twins' comfort between feeds. I advised cutting all wind-forming foods – such as onions, peppers, spices, leeks, chilli, beans and pulses – from her diet for a month.

- Changing the boys' sleep positions: swaddling them at night and making sure they were tucked in securely, with a blanket over their shoulder so they could feel a slight pressure, would make them feel secure. I advised that if the tucking in did not work successfully, the other option would be to swaddle them for daytime naps when sleeping in the cot – a newborn's startle/Moro reflex often wakes them before they are ready to wake naturally.

- Introducing tandem feeding: this would keep the boys on the same routine and cut down the time taken to feed them both. I helped with the logistics of latching on two babies with the rugby-style tandem feeding position and showed Mum how to get set up by preparing bottles before the feed and making sure she had water, muslins and snacks at the feeding area.

- Mixed feeding at each day feed and spacing out their feeding routine to the 7pm–7am routine. Both babies were having 20–30 minutes on the breast and then 60–120ml (2–4oz) from a top-up bottle, ensuring they were both full at each feed and finished within an hour. The 7pm–7am routine also allowed enough time between feeds for their stomachs to empty, longer nap times and longer periods awake.

- Every baby on my routine needs at least 1–2 breasts full of milk at each day feed in order to take enough milk during the day to sleep well and wake less during the night. In order for this to happen with twins, mixed feeding is necessary but the change here is to feed both babies the breast and then immediately top up with expressed breast milk or formula, instead of giving top-ups if and when the breastfeed doesn't satisfy. Feeding the boys at the same time and with the same type of milk would help keep them in sync with each other. Breaking to wind the boys more frequently – at five-minute intervals on the breast and every 30ml (1oz) on the bottle – would help to alleviate wind during and after feeds. This would allow an increase in their milk intake; the less air in their tummies, the more room there is for milk. This increase in milk intake would gradually increase until the boys sleep through the night.

- Introducing the staggered bedtime feed: breastfeed pre-bath for 15–20 minutes, bath, then post-bath bottle. This bottle was introduced at 180ml (6oz) to start with.
- Using the two-minute rule before rushing in to help settle the boys and for night waking. This wasn't actually necessary as both boys responded so well to being fed and winded well, their increased playtime and overall awake time and their new secure sleep positions.

Putting this plan into action resulted in the boys waking once on my first night with them. By the second night they slept through the night, from 8pm to 7am, and they have kept on doing so ever since. Job done in just 48 hours!

12 Steps to 12 Hours' Sleep

M y routine is based around 12 steps that can be used to introduce a simple structure into your baby's life. The steps can be used as a tool to teach a better understanding of my method while following my routine, or they can assist you in creating your own. Maybe your end game isn't a full night's sleep but to help your baby's digestion. Or you need help to encourage better feeding or settling habits. You will find that by following these simple steps they will have a positive effect on your baby's well-being.

Step 1: Start Your Day at the Same Time Every Morning

To encourage routine consistency, and for your day routine to have an effect on your nights, if your baby is not already awake from 6am, wake him up for a 7am feed every morning, regardless of feed timings in the night. This will help set your baby's body clock and allow a flexible routine.

Step 2: Wake Your Baby 10–15 Minutes Before Each Feed

Newborns often find it hard to wake up after a nap and will easily fall asleep again once receiving the comfort of the breast or bottle. Waking your baby 10–15 minutes before each feed and having that time awake, even if it is fractious, will ensure he is wide awake and ready to feed effectively. When breastfeeding it is especially hard for a baby to stay awake while snuggled into Mum as the sucking action alone is soporific. Allowing enough time for your baby to wake properly will help in your quest for active and productive feeding. When your baby reaches 8–10 weeks and becomes interactive, this 10–15 minutes of wake-up time can be used to chat and say hello as, by this stage, your baby will want to communicate and engage with you. Interacting with your baby in this way before a feed means he will be able to focus better on feeding, otherwise you may find that he takes the edge off his hunger and then decides he wants to stop feeding before he is full to chat to you. The result is a reduced milk intake, which has a knock-on effect on your routine and night's sleep.

When teaching your baby the difference between night and day, you need to encourage him to take the majority of his milk and awake time during the day. By waking your baby at specific times you are effectively setting his body clock to eat well at each feed, much like we do as adults, having breakfast, lunch and dinner usually at around the same time every day.

Step 3: Encourage 'Meals' Not Snacks

Making sure your baby is actively feeding, awake and well fed at each feed means you are giving him a 'meal', not a snack that would only sustain him for a short period – an hour or so, maybe less! Offering both breasts at each feed and encouraging active feeding not only stimulates the breasts to make more milk at each feed, but allows your baby to take enough milk to fill him up and sustain him for 3–4 hours. Making sure your baby is full at each feed also encourages longer sleep periods during the day and at night. By slowly and gradually increasing his milk intake during the day, your baby will naturally demand less milk at night, taking the majority of the milk he needs over a 24-hour period during daylight hours. The trick is to allow all feeds to increase but to cap the night feeds: if you are breastfeeding, by 10–15 minutes each side, including winding, and, if you are bottle-feeding, by 120ml (4oz). Over a period of weeks the quantity given at day feeds will become much more substantial than the night feeds, which are phased out naturally at your baby's own pace.

Feeding meals not snacks will enable you to space out your baby's day feeds long enough for his stomach to completely empty before the next feed. This helps aid digestion and overall stomach comfort. Feeding too frequently, every 1–2 hours say, and therefore topping up the stomach with milk before it has had a chance to digest the last feed and empty, causes wind and pain. Feeding too frequently will also inhibit long sleep periods. Once you have established breastfeeding, offer your baby both breasts at each feed for 30 minutes each side (which includes winding) every 3–4 hours during the day and for 15 minutes each side when he naturally wakes at night. When giving a bottle, increase your baby's intake by 15–30ml (½–1oz) per bottle per week until night feeds are phased out and he is sleeping through the night.

As your baby grows, his appetite increases and you'll find that the volume of milk he takes increases dramatically during the first six weeks. Obviously this is hard to gauge while breastfeeding, but expressing should help you understand your milk supply (see page 71). If bottle-feeding, you can easily track your baby's progress.

Active feeding

Active sucking makes for efficient feeding and a well-fed baby. It's so important to teach your baby to associate your breast or the bottle with food, and not with comfort or as an aid for sleep. If you are breastfeeding, this will ultimately increase your milk supply because your breasts are being properly stimulated. Comfort sucking and cat-napping on the breast or bottle leads to less milk intake and disrupted sleep. Comfort sucking looks like a short up-and-down action, often with a shuddery jaw – nibble, nibble, pause, or long pause with the occasional suck. Active feeding looks like a wide circular motion with visible swallowing.

Your baby will naturally slow down as your milk flow slows, but try to encourage him to drain the breast and not slow down until his time is up or your breast is empty (see page 48 for how to check your breasts for milk). Allow 30 minutes for each breast, including winding, until your flow of milk speeds up, your baby becomes an efficient feeder and he is sleeping through the night – this will happen at around Weeks 4–8. If you have a lower milk supply you may need to shorten the time on each breast to 20 minutes and top up if necessary in order to achieve longer periods of sleep at night. Help by massaging each breast while your baby is feeding for the last five minutes of the feed – it's all about teamwork! That said, it is hard for a newborn baby to stay awake while feeding. In the first weeks of life, the sucking action alone is tiring and the cuddle-like position of breastfeeding is comforting.

A build-up of wind, which gives a false sense of fullness, slowed milk flow and falling asleep all cause comfort sucking.

Bottle-fed babies tend to be more active when feeding than breastfed babies due to the constant flow of milk, but they can still start to doze off and lose focus. Drinking milk too quickly and finishing their bottle of milk in less than 30 minutes can result in a milk slump, vomiting and an inability to wake up. Wind regularly, at 15–30ml (½–1oz) intervals and use your spare hand to prompt him to keep your baby actively sucking. Don't allow dozing and comfort sucking which is bad for digestion and leads to ineffective feeding.

Top tips for active feeding

1. Keep the room cool for feeding and awake time during the day (19–20°C ideally) and strip your baby down to a vest bodysuit only. Creating a positive, calm and quiet environment for feeding will help your baby to stay awake.
2. Whenever feeding hits a prolonged pause, use your free hand to tickle your baby's chin, ears, feet and body to prompt him so he doesn't drift off to sleep and starts sucking again.
3. Break for frequent winding. A baby under six weeks old will not be able to remain actively breastfeeding for more than 5–10 minutes at a time. A bottle-fed baby will need a break every 15–30ml (½–1oz). As soon as sucking starts to slow and prompts are no longer working, break to wake your baby, wind him and allow him time to regain focus.

4. When breastfeeding use a good feeding pillow like the 'My Brest Friend' or 'Doomoo' feeding pillows. When bottle-feeding, place your baby on a pillow or cushion in front of you while feeding, rather than cuddling him in your arms. For twin feeding, using a pillow like the 'Peanut & Piglet' can work brilliantly for smaller, high breasts. Two square, firm bed pillows work well for larger breasts and tandem bottle-feeding (see page 146).

5. Always remember that feeding is for food intake, not for cuddling your baby to sleep. Instead have your snuggle time before his naps, when he wakes from a nap or even during a nap with skin-on-skin contact (see page 197).

Step 4: Focus on Winding and Digestion

Your baby's digestive comfort will affect every part of your routine and is key to its success and a full night's sleep. Newborns are unable to burp themselves and only become able to self-wind at around 8–12 weeks of age. It is hugely underestimated how much newborn babies need to be winded in order to be comfortable to feed, play and sleep well. Winding your baby frequently is very important as air in the tummy can swell up, giving a false sense of fullness, which makes a baby feel sleepy and can keep your baby asleep until the wind is relieved. This will not only lead to hunger (and therefore disrupted sleep) as your baby will not have fed enough, but it will also make him feel sleepy. The trapped wind can cause pain when the air travels through your baby's digestive system, which, in turn, will also make for unsettled sleep. Trapped wind can also cause vomiting as the milk sits on top of a big air bubble in the stomach and, when you do eventually get the air out, it often brings the milk back up – this is known as 'posseting' (see page 11). I should say that a posset alone, which can happen often during and after a feed, does not mean your baby has wind, but babies will often posset milk when a burp pushes milk up on its way out.

I find that babies on my routine rarely pass wind. This is because my routine encourages you to expel most of the air caused by feeding throughout and after feeds through regular winding. In the first six weeks of life you will need to wind your baby every 5–10 minutes on the breast and every 15–30ml (½–1oz) on the bottle. Once you have finished feeding, your baby is still digesting milk, which creates gas, so you will need to wind him 10–15 minutes after feeding and then again 15–20 minutes after the last burp. This should come up easily, but if not check again in another 10–15 minutes. Don't spend any length of time over this extra winding. Likewise, the winding process during feeds should take no longer than a few minutes – don't spend most of the feed time winding. If you are breastfeeding and your milk is fast-flowing from around Week 4 then break to wind at two-minute intervals for the first two wind breaks on each breast.

To wind your baby make sure he is awake as you cannot wind a sleeping baby. Sit your baby on your knee with one of your hands supporting his stomach up to the chest so he has a nice straight back, with your forefinger and thumb supporting his chin and head. Pat his back with your other hand, cupping and moulding your hand around his back. By moulding your hand you are not directly patting his spine but either side of it. Rub his back using firm, circular, upward strokes.

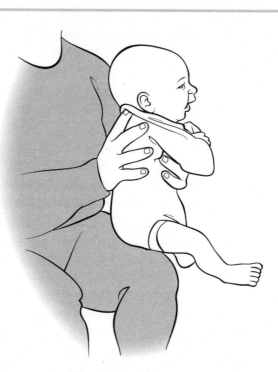

Winding your baby on the knee

It's a myth that breastfed babies do not need winding; breastfed babies are as windy as bottle-fed babies! A baby drinks, therefore he has wind. Certain foods, such as the onion family and spices, can add fuel to the fire with wind issues so try and avoid these wind-forming foods in the first six weeks if you are breastfeeding.

You will find that effective winding makes all the difference to how long your baby sleeps. The less air in his tummy, the more milk he can take on and the happier playtime and better quality sleep he will have. Not winding frequently enough and effectively is the most common problem I come across with unsettled babies and sleep issues.

Step 5: Establish Structured Awake/ Playtime After Feeds

Contrary to popular belief, babies do much more than just feeding and sleeping in the first three months of life. Most babies in my care, aged 1–2 weeks old, are able to stay awake for 1¼–2 hours at each feed period, enjoying black-and-white pictures, looking around and working out their new environment. The aim is to keep your baby active and awake during and after feeds, while he digests the milk feed, though you will find that it is common for babies to become soporific during this period. Encouraging awake time helps with digestion by making sure your baby is wind-free before bed and nap time.

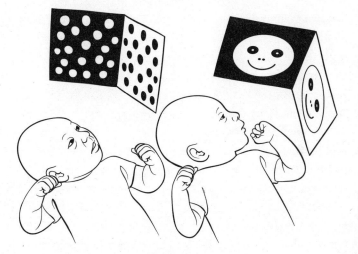

Stimulating tummy time

Having just been fed, this is also the most content time for your baby to be awake, which enables you to work out if he has had enough milk. A well-fed and winded baby will be able to play happily and engage. By encouraging

161

awake time after feeds you are also teaching your baby the difference between night and day, which naturally has a positive effect on your nights.

Your baby's awake time should be increased gradually over the first six weeks of life. With every baby in my care I first work out what each baby is capable of, by how long they regularly and naturally stay awake for after a feed, and build on that time. Of course, this may need to be helped along by a reviving nappy change after a feed to get your baby to wake if he has fallen asleep on the breast or bottle. Keep encouraging a longer awake time until each feed period is two hours. For some babies in my care this happens at Week 2, while for others it is at Weeks 4–6.

It's important to recognise that your baby is not a robot and, during growth spurts, he may need more sleep and find it harder to stay awake. The aim is to encourage awake time at each feed period and, as sleep improves at night and your baby gets older, the easier he will find it to stay awake. Make sure you are starting your feeds and playtime somewhere you can remain still for the duration, such as at your house, or a friend or family member's home. Newborns are unable to stay awake during motion and will quickly fall asleep while being pushed in the pram, driven in the car or worn in a sling. They will also struggle to stay awake if a room is too noisy or warm. It's important for the routine that your baby falls asleep when he is truly tired, and not because of digestion, trapped wind or being coaxed into sleep with a cuddle, in a car seat or in the pram, which will make for unsettled sleep.

To help keep your little one awake:

- Change his nappy after each day feed to help revive him for playtime. A tepid water bottom wash works best.

- Engage your baby with black-and-white pictures. Make your own with a black marker pen or 'My Social Baby' has some great black-and-white face and pattern books. Lay your baby on a play mat with pictures in his eyeline. Make sure you don't overwhelm him with lots of pictures and toys – he will need to focus and single out images.
- Make sure your baby is cool, keeping the room temperature between 19°C and 20°C where possible. Babies are heat-sensitive and a few degrees over 20°C will make it a struggle to stay awake. A baby's body temperature will rise when feeding and digesting milk, which again makes a baby feel sleepy. This, of course, is not due to tiredness so it is important to understand the difference, making sure your baby falls asleep when he is actually tired and not when he is too warm or in a milk slumber. Be consistent with attempts to routinely wake your baby after a feed – if he is actually tired you will not be able to wake him, but often, with some encouragement, he will ping awake.
- Choose a quiet room for playtime. Background noise, such as the TV, washing machine, radio or vacuum cleaner, can lull your baby to sleep. Most newborns are sensitive to noise, so use your voice only to stimulate him in the first 3–6 weeks.
- Keep the lights low. Overhead spotlights or bright sunlight will keep your baby's eyes shut. With very poor vision most babies need a low-lit room and start to handle bright light from six weeks old.
- Make sure that structured awake/playtime is indoors and not in motion. A baby will not stay awake being pushed outside in the pram. Being pushed around after a feed is bad for your baby's digestion and will

send him to sleep, but not because he is tired. Investing time in feeding your baby and giving stimulating play will have a positive effect on your nights.

Step 6: Teach Positive Associations with Self-settling

Putting your baby down to sleep while he is still awake will teach self-settling. In the first few weeks this may be tricky as your baby may fall asleep while you are encouraging playtime or as soon as you start cuddling him. Once he is able to stay awake for two hours and is still awake just before his nap, then you can make sure he is put down to bed still awake but calmed and cuddled to encourage self-settling. Rocking or cuddling your baby to sleep is teaching him to associate falling asleep in this way. At some point, when he is a bit older, you will want him to settle himself and he won't be able to. Teaching positive associations from the start is much kinder than having to break habits and cause confusion later on.

Having met all your baby's needs – a full tummy, winded and sufficient awake time – he should settle easily without the aid of rocking, cuddling, a dummy or being pushed in the pram. If he does not settle you will need to work out why. Is he still hungry? Does he have wind? Has he not had enough awake time? Is he not swaddled and tucked into a pram or cot?

Despite the importance of teaching your baby to self-settle, you need to ensure you have a balance and allow plenty of cuddle and skin-on-skin time with your baby. This will ensure that you are getting the much-needed recovery rest which will help increase your milk supply and provide the all-important emotional bonding. Try to allocate one nap every day, or every other day, for skin-on-skin naps where your baby can sleep on you naked (but, of course, leave his nappy on!). See page 197 for more on skin-on-skin naps. If you feel you need extra cuddles, pick your baby up from a nap and cuddle him 10–20 minutes earlier than your usual 10–15 minutes wake up, before feeds.

Naps should otherwise be in your baby's bedroom in a cot, Moses basket or the pram, and he should be tucked in. Tucking your baby into bed will provide him with a feeling of comfort, being cuddled and security. (See Chapter Thirteen for more on sleep positions and tucking in.) Letting your baby fall asleep on a play mat or in a baby chair will not encourage good sleep habits.

Step 7: Swaddle Your Baby

Swaddling makes a baby feel secure and cuddled; it is the only prop I use to aid peaceful sleep. Babies go through much more light sleep periods than we do as adults and also have a startle ('Moro') reflex, which tends to kick in at around 3–6 weeks of age. The startle reflex means that a baby's arms have no control and will startle and wave around, which can often wake a baby. Once woken, he will often find it hard to get back to sleep. Babies need to feel secure in order to sleep so swaddling at night and being tucked into their bed aids peaceful sleep.

If you find your baby's day naps are unsettled then use the swaddle for day naps as well. I will usually swaddle a baby until they are sleeping through the night for a full two weeks, then wean them off by taking the swaddle away during the day for a week and then half-swaddling with one arm out at night for a few nights, before taking it awake completely by 4–5 months old. If it's too soon for your baby and he is unsettled without the swaddle, keep swaddling for another two weeks and then try again. There is no need to rush the process.

Sleep positions are also important for enabling peaceful sleep (see page 199). I often see mothers pushing their wailing babies around in prams. Nine out of ten times the babies are flat on their backs with no covers on or with their arms flailing about. Babies need to feel secure in order to sleep. Tuck a blanket tightly over your baby's shoulders and arms wherever he sleeps, as well as using the swaddle at night and if needed for day naps. Keep your baby's blankets tucked in well to the sides of the pram, cot or Moses basket and at shoulder height so the material is not around your baby's face. Loose blankets can be dangerous and can cause suffocation.

Though government advice is to sleep babies on their backs, and not on their stomachs or sides so they cannot roll on to their stomachs, I sleep babies slightly tilted on their sides using a roll pillow, which means they are unable to roll on to their stomachs. With the roll pillow, your baby's back is leaning slightly raised on the pillow so any movement will result in back sleeping if used properly. If you wish to try side sleeping with your baby, discuss this with a healthcare professional first, and please see the video on my website for how to use roll pillows safely: www.thesleepingbabyroutine.co.uk. I change the direction the baby faces every 24 hours to form a perfectly round head and to eliminate the risk of flat head syndrome.

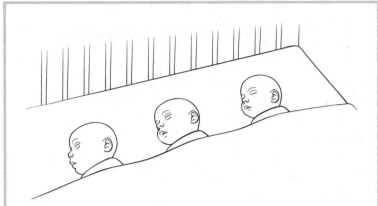

Three babies tucked in securely

As the swaddling material and roll pillows (if using) can often raise your baby's body slightly higher than his head, always raise the head of the cot, pram or Moses basket slightly higher than the feet. Use a rolled-up muslin under the Moses basket mattress or a small blanket under the cot mattress to ever so slightly raise the angle. Also ensure that you place your baby in the 'feet to foot' position, where his feet are at the end of the cot, Moses basket or pram. Please see the video on my website for how to safely swaddle your baby: www.thesleepingbabyroutine.co.uk.

Step 8: Change Your Baby's Nappy After Each Daytime Feed

Changing your baby's nappy after each daytime feed has two benefits:

1. A baby usually fills his nappy during feeds so the nappy is more likely to be full after a feed.
2. The nappy change can be used as a tool to wake your baby up for playtime.

These days, quality disposable nappies work so well drawing moisture away from babies' bottoms that nappy rash is not usually an issue. The key is to keep your baby's bottom dry. Use plain, unbleached white kitchen roll to blot your baby's bottom dry before putting on a fresh nappy. You shouldn't need to use a barrier cream unless nappy rash occurs. Nappy rash is usually a result of poor hygiene, not drying a baby's bottom properly after changing, the mother's diet (too much acidity), teething or using low-grade, cheaper nappies which don't absorb as well as the leading brands. If you are using lower-grade, eco-friendly nappies, you will need to change your baby before and after each daytime feed to keep him dry and prevent a sore, red bottom. If you need to change your baby's nappy before a day feed then change it after the feed as well.

In terms of changing your baby at night-time, I recommend changing his nappy *before* a feed. Changing your baby before a night-time feed will avoid stimulation just before you want to settle him back to sleep. In fact, if your baby is only waking once in the night, you may not need to change his nappy at all, unless it is dirty of course.

Your baby's body clock soon learns the difference between night and day and he will stop pooing at night usually when he starts sleeping through the night. I would highly recommend using a leading brand, such as Pampers Baby Dry, for night-time sleep; other nappies simply will not keep your baby's bottom as dry. Some nappies now have a blue line indicator to let you know when your baby is wet. However, this *does not* mean that you need to change your baby's nappy. Babies constantly wee and if you were to change his nappy every time a blue line showed you would be changing your baby three times more often than you need to. In my opinion, this wetness indicator is just a clever tactic by nappy companies to make you use and buy more nappies! You might want to try using a larger size nappy at night to absorb more and enable a longer time between nappy changes once your baby is sleeping through the night, but make sure the nappy is fitted securely around the legs to prevent any leaks.

If your baby has woken early or is unsettled during sleep for any reason, changing his nappy will only stimulate him! I have never known a baby to be upset and woken due to a wet or dirty nappy. It's often thought that a nappy change will calm a baby and they will settle to sleep again once dry. However, in my experience, this will not work – your baby has woken or is crying for another reason and the nappy change will only stimulate and wake him fully, rather than soothe him back to sleep.

Step 9: Establish a Bedtime Routine

Staggering your baby's last feed of the day and splitting it with a bath, whether you are breast- or bottle-feeding, will help to make this feed the largest and most important of all the daytime feeds, which will be key to helping your baby sleep for longer overnight. By staggering your baby's milk intake and offering only a small amount of milk, including winding, before the bath helps for a calm bath without your baby screaming for milk. This really must be a small amount of milk: a maximum of 60ml (2oz) from the bottle or 10–15 minutes from each breast. Too much milk at this time may cause vomiting on the post-bath feed, from being sloshed around in the bath with a full tummy. Your baby may object to such a restricted feed at this time, but rest assured he will soon recognise it as part of the routine. Slow the 60ml (2oz) feed by breaking every 15ml (½oz), walk your baby around to distract him, or take him into the bathroom while you run the bath – the sound of running water has a white noise calming effect. Splitting the feed with the bath will enable your baby to take the majority of his milk after the bath, close to bedtime, and will mean he is ready to settle for a full night's sleep or his longest stretch of sleep. Giving a bath as part of your bedtime routine also helps your baby to recognise that bedtime/night-time is coming. In the first six weeks while establishing the routine it's a stimulating part of the day and your baby's fourth awake period of the day.

Your baby's bath temperature should be quite cool at the newborn stage – 34°C, or 32°C if we are in a heatwave and 35°C if it's arctic weather! Use a bath thermometer, like the Philips AVENT bath and room thermometer, not your hand or elbow as we all have variations in skin sensitivity. As I mentioned earlier, babies are heat-sensitive, so a bath that is too warm will send your baby to sleep quickly and before he has had a chance to finish his bedtime feed. Only when your baby is out of the newborn stage, from three months old, will he be less heat-sensitive, so the temperature of the bath can increase. By this time you can also use the bath time routine as a calming, soothing tool to help settle your baby at bedtime and you can increase the duration of the bath as your baby finds the experience much more fun.

There is no need to actually wash your baby with soap every day – a sloshing of water for 5–10 minutes will do. For those newborns who are not yet used to the bath, make sure they are always covered in water by sloshing water over their tummies. I use a bath support, such as Angelcare, which goes into the bath and means you don't have to break your back over the bath. These will usually last up until you use a seated position. Never step away from the bath – using a bath support may be hands-free, but you should never leave your baby unattended in water. A baby's eye ducts are not working in the first 4–6 weeks of life – you may have noticed that your newborn does not cry tears – so any water or particles that get into the eyes are unable to drain away. For this reason, try not to get water into your baby's eyes during bath time in the early days.

Introduce a bedtime bottle at Week 2

If you are breastfeeding, regardless of your milk supply, your milk will naturally deplete throughout the day. You can boost your supply with a lunchtime skin-on-skin nap, by resting, expressing or through your diet, but inevitably your supply will be lower in the late afternoon/evening than the morning. You may, in the first few weeks, have enough milk to satisfy your baby for the last and biggest feed of the day, but as your baby's appetite grows to full capacity in 6–8 weeks, you will naturally have your lowest supply in the evenings. A poor design by Mother Nature indeed! If you are looking to get a full night's sleep and phase out night waking, introducing a bottle of expressed breast milk, collected throughout the day, or formula at the last feed of the day will give your baby the boost and milk needed to sleep through the night. This bottle is key to the success of my routine. Babies at this time of day can be very sleepy and hard to feed so not only does the bottle-feed enable you to give a big feed but you won't have the added issue of your baby drifting off to sleep as much as he would on the breast before he is full.

Another reason for introducing the bottle in the first weeks of life is that you won't come up against bottle refusal. Rest assured, the bottle is your friend and this one bottle a day will not interfere with breastfeeding. Your baby will not reject your breast because of it or be confused, but instead will recognise it as part of his bedtime routine. This bottle-feed will result in a well-fed baby who sleeps for long periods at night. If you introduce a bottle at a later stage it may be, and often is, rejected. Introducing a bottle early on is also handy if, as a breastfeeding mother, you ever get sick, your supply dips or your baby is sick and throws up all his milk. If you don't have enough breast milk collected giving formula at this stage is a win–win as your baby has all the night benefits of breast milk, and supplementing with formula at this time of day can often help babies sleep longer as it is heavier in composition and sustains for longer. This bottle-feed is a very small percentage of your baby's overall milk intake and using formula at this time has no disadvantages. You should gradually increase the amount of this bottle-feed by 15–30ml (½–1oz) at a time until your baby has reached his own personal number of ounces needed to sleep through the night. I have found over the last 20 years that this number is generally between 200ml (7oz) and 260ml (9oz), which is usually reached between four and eight weeks of age. Bottle, teat shape and size do matter so head back to the bottle-feeding chapter to learn more (page 102).

Step 10: Baby-led Nights

Once you have established breastfeeding and your baby has regained his birth weight, is over 2.72kg (6lb) and is gaining weight, which should all happen by around Week 2, in contrast to your day routine you should let your baby wake of his own accord for feeds at night. This is where my technique differs from other baby experts who advise waking your baby on the dot for each feed day and night, or waking him for a 'dream feed' (a booster feed which is given before the parent would naturally go to bed). On my routine your nights are 'baby-led': if your baby is hungry, he will wake for a feed at night. By encouraging the majority of your baby's milk intake during the day, combined with the staggered feed and bottle at bedtime, there is no need to wake your baby for a dream feed. As your baby's day feeds and awake time increase over the weeks so will the length of time he sleeps at night, getting the much-needed rest to grow and thrive. As a result your baby will learn the difference between night and day very early on and night feeds will become efficient and short. You will also get the much-needed rest you need to recover and take care of your new baby.

When breastfeeding your baby will get into a routine much quicker than your breast, which can leave you feeling full, uncomfortable and unable to last until your baby naturally wakes. Your breasts will also need extra stimulation to make up for the loss of stimulation from your baby as he sleeps longer at night at this early stage. To combat this, express before you go to bed for the night at around 8–9pm. This will not only help keep your supply tip-top but keep you comfortable until your baby wakes naturally.

Top tips for night feeding

- Keep your baby's room dark, using blackout blinds in the summer, and with no night light. Keep the camera monitor light covered as it will shine straight on to your baby's face. Once he has reached six weeks and wakes in the night, any light, albeit dim lighting, will stimulate him. Night lights can be used, if at all, much later on, at around six months plus.

- Keep night feeds in the same room as your baby sleeps in. Moving rooms, turning lights on and walking around are stimulating and will encourage waking. Practise short, dark, quiet feeds with no talking, phones or TV.

- Swaddle your baby at night until he is sleeping through the night for at least two weeks. If he wakes and the swaddle is loose or his arms have come out, this may be the only reason for waking and he will not be able to resettle with his arms waving around. Re-swaddle him, give him a cuddle and then pop him back to bed. Regardless of the reason for waking, a newborn will immediately think 'milk', so you may need to feed him if re-swaddling and reset-tling doesn't work. The swaddle technique is key to your baby settling! Tuck him into bed with no loose blankets. Babies feel secure, cuddled and sleep better if they are wrapped and firmly tucked in. This also helps to stop him waking due to the startle reflex. (See page 165 and Chapter Thirteen for more advice on swaddling and tucking in.)

- Change your baby's nappy *before* night feeds. Changing his nappy after a feed will again stimulate him and encourage waking, making it more difficult for him to settle back to sleep.

- Night feeds should take no longer than 30 minutes, regardless of whether you are breast- or bottle-feeding. The idea is to change your baby, feed him and then put him back to bed quickly. The length and quantity of feeds should decrease the later your baby wakes. This is to help phase out night feeds and to not interfere with the morning feed at 7am. The maximum for any one night feed is capped at 30 minutes or 120ml (4oz) from a bottle. When breastfeeding, the later your baby wakes the more milk you have and the less time needed to feed.

- 10pm–3am: 30 minutes (15 minutes each side) or 120ml (4oz) from a bottle, including winding, less if your baby wants
- 3am–4am: 20 minutes (10 minutes each side) or 90ml (3oz) from a bottle, including winding
- 4am–5am: 10 minutes (5 minutes each side) or 60ml (2oz) from a bottle, including winding and keep your baby swaddled. No nappy change (if possible)
- 5am–6am: No feed zone. If your baby has slept all the way through until 5am or 6am, he has slept the majority of the night so feeding at this time will be stimulating and he will most likely want a breakfast feed, not a snack, to get back to sleep. Feeding at this time will dramatically interfere with the 7am feed which can have a knock-on effect on your whole day routine. If your baby wakes at this time, keep him swaddled and cuddle him back to sleep by holding him on your chest firmly (cover up any naked skin which will only frustrate and not calm your baby – use a muslin or pop a top on), patting his back and bottom, and breathing deeply. This is a form of the 'shush and hold' technique (see page 205). As a very last resort, let your baby suck on your finger which will calm and soothe him. Stay in your baby's bedroom or go back to your bed in the dark. Start your day at 6am and switch your routine to the four-hourly 6am routine that day.

This is the only time of day I would advise letting your baby suck your finger or cuddling your baby back to sleep as I don't believe in babies sucking for comfort. It creates wind and has a negative effect on the morning feed.

- Swaddle your baby for the last five minutes of the night feed and let him drift to sleep, winding him over your shoulder and then promptly putting him back to bed.

Step 11: Wait Two Minutes for Your Baby to Resettle

The 'two-minute rule' applies night and day, waiting two minutes to see if your baby resettles himself back to sleep. Babies wake often and go through many light periods of sleep. Most babies wake, shout and fall back to sleep until they are actually ready to be fed. You must allow your baby to do this to help encourage self-settling. This also means you are not jumping to his every whim, stimulating your baby awake unnecessarily or getting him up to feed when he is not ready. Babies who are picked up as soon as they shout, soon learn this is how to get picked up and you will end up with a baby who cries more, is insecure and is unable to be put down or settle himself.

The two-minute rule is not controlled crying but is instead simply a short pause to check and make sure your baby truly needs your attention. Babies cry! It's their only way of verbal communication. It does not always mean they need feeding or attention. Babies cry to settle themselves, on waking, due to wind or when they are hungry. Giving your baby two minutes before you help him out will teach confidence in you and your baby's ability to self-settle. The two-minute rule is for crying, not squeaking or grunting which most babies do in their sleep. Time it to make sure you are not jumping to attention too quickly.

The only time you would not wait for two minutes is after the bedtime feed. This is the only time of day your baby will go to bed on a full stomach. With the day feeds, he has playtime to digest his feeds and the night feeds are much lighter. If your baby cries out after you have settled him to bed, it is likely to be due to wind, overstimulation or because he is still hungry. Firstly, check for wind and then that the swaddle is secure. Give your baby a calming cuddle over the shoulder, in a dark or a very dimly-lit room, and if he still doesn't settle, offer another 30–60ml (1–2oz) of milk. The last 30ml (1oz) should be slow moving, so if he finishes the bottle easily, offer a little more and increase it by another ounce the following evening.

Step 12: Be Flexible with Your Routine

The 7pm to 7am Sleeping Baby Routine allows your routine to be flexible. Your growing baby is not a robot and will often wake early or you may simply need to change the routine according to your day. Having said this, all my variations of the routine end the day with the same timings for the bath and bedtime routine. Ending each day at the same time encourages consistency which is important for your baby to recognise that bedtime is coming and to set his body clock to sleep at night.

Below are some alternative routine feed timings:

- 6am, 10am, 2pm, 6pm pre-bath feed, 6.30pm bath, 6.45pm bottle, 7.30pm bed

- 6.30am, 10/10.30am, 2/2.30pm, 6pm pre-bath feed, 6.30pm bath, 6.45pm bottle, 7.30pm bed
- 7am, 10.30/11am, 2.30pm, 6pm pre-bath feed, 6.30pm bath, 6.45pm bottle, 7.30pm bed
- 7am, 11am, 2.30/3pm, 6pm pre-bath feed, 6.30pm bath, 6.45pm bottle, 7.30pm bed
- 7.30am, 11/11.30am, 3pm, 6pm pre-bath feed, 6.30pm bath, 6.45pm bottle, 7.30pm bed

These 12 steps will help you to understand your baby's needs and give you the flexibility if your routine goes a little off-piste. A routine needs to be flexible but consistent for it to work during the newborn stage, but once you are established everything becomes much less restrictive and automatic, and you will have a happy, sleeping baby.

PART FOUR

Work, Rest and Play

Chapter Eleven

Your Health and Recovery

L ooking after yourself physically and mentally after having a baby is of the utmost importance at this often emotional and sleep-deprived time of life. Becoming a parent is a wonderful life-changing experience. For the first 2–4 weeks you will either ride high on adrenalin with all the excitement and love you feel for the life you have created, or you will feel completely overwhelmed and anxious with the responsibility of this new life you have created … Sorry, I'm just being honest! Either way these new emotions, the sleep deprivation and recovering from the birth can mean, if you don't look after yourself, you can hit a brick wall at around Weeks 3–5. Physically this can lead to exhaustion and, if you are breastfeeding, a low milk supply and the risk of infections such as mastitis. Mentally this can leave you with the baby blues, a low mood or, worst case, postnatal depression.

My routine will help you with sleep deprivation as it encourages long periods of sleep during the day and night. As I have said in previous chapters, your body is firstly using energy to recover from the birth, secondly for daily activity and lastly for lactation, so when breastfeeding it's doubly important to rest, nap during the day, go to bed early – until your baby is at least waking only once in the night – and eat well.

Make time to look after yourself – eat between feeds and don't even contemplate a diet yet if you are breastfeeding. Plan your meals so that they are prepared before you start feeding your baby and, if you can and you are reading this while you are pregnant, fill the freezer up with home-made, ready-to-go meals. Remember when breastfeeding to leave out the wind-forming foods I mentioned on page 34.

You may not feel like you need to sleep or rest during the day but it's important that you do. Go to bed early – ideally at around 9pm but before 10pm – until your baby is sleeping through the night so you aim to get 7–8 hours' sleep overall. A happy mum makes for a happy baby, so looking after yourself during the newborn stage will mean you are giving your baby the best start. Aim to have one skin-on-skin nap a day, or at least every other day, to support your newborn's emotional development (see page 197 for more on this).

Low mood

During the first month of sleep deprivation and hormonal changes, having a baby is not always glamorous and I find that even mothers in a group like the NCT will not discuss how they are feeling and what's actually going on with their bodies. The reality is that you will experience one or all of the symptoms of your body changing, the most common being mood swings and crying for no reason, known as the 'baby blues'. This is not postnatal depression and often letting the tears fall and talking to your family will make you feel better until the next wave of emotion. A mother carries her baby for nine months and gives birth, and then, while recovering from that, has to get up in the night, sometimes several times. However, that doesn't take away from the fact that becoming a parent is a huge, life-changing experience which affects both parents. It's common for dads to also feel the pressure and emotions that surround this huge change. Dads can feel the responsibility financially as well as emotionally as they adjust to their new role, maybe feeling like they are missing out while out at work all day, only to come back to a tired partner. At times they may think they need to take a back seat and feel less involved, especially if Mum is breastfeeding. For both parents, these moments will pass as you get used to your new baby, but it's natural to feel the pressure and responsibility for the new life you have created.

Postnatal depression can be triggered by lack of sleep. If you are susceptible to depression, it can run in the family and come on at any point during the first year after birth. Holding your feelings in and putting on a brave face is not a healthy way forward and certainly with postnatal depression you must seek help. Be open with friends, family members, midwives and health visitors with how you are feeling. Being open will enable you to form a plan to address the problem and help you on a quicker road to feeling like yourself again.

Anxiety

Anxiety and tension may stop you sleeping even when your baby is sleeping. The anticipation of your baby waking can cause tension and lack of sleep which affects your mood and milk supply. Have a good cry if you need to, watch a sad film and let it all out with your feet up; *Marley and Me* gets me every time! Make time to relax before bed and create a calming, positive environment to encourage sleep. Drops of lavender oil in a warm bath or on your pillow can help with relaxation. Cut out caffeine and instead drink herbal night tea before bed, such as Pukka's Night Time Tea which contains lavender and oat flower. Read instead of using your phone, tablet or the TV to relax you. If your anxiety and low mood does not lift, discuss your feelings with friends, family, health visitors or your GP.

Anxiety can also affect your let-down when breastfeeding as holding tension in your neck, back, hips, legs and shoulders can stop you releasing milk. Make sure you sit in a good feeding position and use a breastfeeding pillow for support so you are not using your arms (see page 41). This will also help to keep baby awake when feeding. The 'My Brest Friend' or 'Doomoo' feeding pillows are my go-to pillows. If you are breastfeeding you may feel discomfort through your nipples in the early days, which only adds to the tension. Squeeze your shoulders up to your ears and then release the tension. I also find a microwaveable heated wheat bag helps around the shoulders before you start feeding to help relieve any tension. It's also a good idea to use a firm pillow or cushion when bottle-feeding (to support your baby instead of in your arm which sends tension through the arm, up to the shoulder and to your neck and back). This makes for easy, hands-free, back-supporting feeding – see page 107.

Night sweats

Night sweats are another taboo topic it seems, but they are a normal symptom of recovery. Night sweats are simply a result of your hormones pushing out the extra fluid that you needed during pregnancy, which can take weeks of on–off sweating. Night sweats can leave you feeling like you've just stepped out of the shower and can lead to a soaked bed. Have a change of bed clothes by the side of the bed and sleep on a towel with an extra sheet between you and the duvet, so when you wake up feeling soggy, you can quickly change and strip the sheet and towel away leaving you nice and dry again.

Afterpains

Afterpains are a cramping feeling as your uterus contracts. Afterpains can be intensified while breastfeeding, but this is a good sign as, although uncomfortable, it means your uterus is shrinking. Afterpains are generally more painful with each baby you have, due to poorer muscle tone.

Memory loss

'Baby brain' or memory loss is common but it is just your hormones playing you up again. The fog will pass eventually, but it can be exacerbated by sleep deprivation. Write everything down and keep a baby diary as even remembering which breast you started on at the last feed can be challenging (see page 50 for more on this). There are, of course, apps to keep track of your baby's feeds and sleep times, but using your own diary allows you to write down specifics about her behaviour and awake time, as well as any winding details.

Visitors

You may be inundated with flowers and visitors during the first few weeks, which is lovely but may leave you feeling exhausted having constantly entertained friends and family. The subsequent loss of focus on your baby's feeds and her routine may result in an unsettled baby. Visitors often tend to not understand how it feels during the early establishing stage, even if they have children themselves, as this time is intense for you but is a short period of your life which is easily forgotten by everyone else.

Don't feel like you need to entertain your visitors; they should be bringing you lunch and snacks and making you cups of fennel tea, not the other way round. Allocate a specific time of day for visitors, and state when that time is and why. For example, if you ask people to visit at 12.30pm, you will have finished feeding, winding and expressing and your baby will be having playtime and then a nap. End the visit at 1.30pm which will give you time to have a rest before the next feed. Meet friends out for a walk or in a café during one of your baby's nap times. This will limit your meeting to your baby's nap time only, getting you out and back home for her next feed. You need to focus on your feeds during the first two months, which take up to an hour with effective winding and structured awake time after in order for your baby to digest her milk. This needs to be in the right environment (see page 188). Rest assured this all changes once you and your baby are established.

You must put you and your baby, and your health, first above anyone else's feelings at this stage. Once feeding is established, you have recovered from the birth, your baby is sleeping through the night and you have got your routine going, you will have plenty of time to entertain friends and family.

Chapter Twelve

Structured Awake Time and Stimulation

I t's generally thought that, in the first three months of life, a newborn will do nothing but feed and sleep. In my experience this is just not so; some babies of only one week old can stay awake for up to two hours during a feed period, checking out their surroundings and trying to focus on Mum's face, and black-and-white objects or pictures.

In the first month, your baby can only see a short distance of 20–30cm (8–12in) away and prefers looking at black-and-white objects or images. It is easy to make your own pictures using a black marker pen on white paper. Of course, his favourite object to look at will be your face. Too many toys to look at at one time will be confusing, so don't overcrowd – show him only one or two pictures at a time. Black-and-white pictures and toys need to be static until your baby is able to track and follow them at around Weeks 6–8. He won't be able to focus on moving mobiles or toys until this time but he will be greatly stimulated by your voice and touch. High-pitched noises and tones of voice work a treat to get a reaction. Cooing and copying your baby's sounds encourages communication and will be more stimulating than your normal tone of voice.

The length of time babies can stay awake in the early days will vary from baby to baby. Your baby's awake time may even vary at each playtime and from day to day as he grows and has growth spurts. Encouraging a steadily increasing awake time during each feed period helps to ensure a good night's sleep for you all as well as good daytime naps for your baby. I generally work out what a newborn is personally capable of, usually 1¼–2 hours of awake time at each feed period, and then increase and build on that until the baby reaches a full two hours at each feed period by Weeks 4–6. Your baby's total awake time should include feeding, winding, playtime and settling.

The right environment

To encourage successful awake time during the day you need to create the right environment for your newborn who will be very sensitive to heat, motion, light and noise. Newborns are extremely heat-sensitive, so the room temperature and weather can affect your baby's wakefulness. Just a few degrees over 20°C is enough to make it hard for most newborns to wake and stay awake. The ideal room temperature for awake time is between 19°C and 20°C. Your newborn's body will also heat up while he is feeding and digesting milk, again making it hard for him to wake up for playtime. Strip your baby down to his vest bodysuit only for all day feeds and when trying to wake him for playtime. It's normal for your baby's hands and feet to be cool – feel his body for an accurate body temperature.

Newborns are also light-sensitive; if the lights are too bright your baby won't be able to open his eyes. The level of sensitivity obviously varies from newborn to newborn, but generally a baby under six weeks of age will not be able to open his eyes in daylight when taken outside, and will automatically fall asleep. This is another reason why all awake periods must be indoors and to only venture outside in the pram, car seat or sling during nap times. When a baby is looking up from the floor while lying on a play mat or feeding, the glare of overhead spotlights especially will make it hard for him to keep his eyes open. The same is true for the sun streaming in through a window. Try to keep your baby's playtime and feeds in a dimmed light to make it easier for him to see. It's normal for newborns to feed with their eyes shut but once shut they will soon start to fall asleep. Keeping your baby awake during feeds and awake time will encourage solid sleep during naps and at night.

Newborns are unable to distinguish colour for the first four weeks, with bold colours like red and yellow becoming visible by 4–6 weeks of age. Black and white are the most stimulating colours in the first two months of your baby's life. Shaded dimly-lit rooms are ideal for babies to be able to focus, thus stimulating and engaging the brain to help keep them awake. Test your baby's light sensitivity by drawing a curtain or leaving the lights off during the day to see if he finds it easier to open his eyes. Having said this, it is important if your baby has jaundice that he is exposed to natural light: give your baby a nap in the pram so he is exposed to natural light, or place his Moses basket close to the window, once a day for the first few weeks until he has been signed off by the midwife (be careful that the sun is not directly on your baby's face). Upping your own vitamin D intake – supplementing with a vitamin D oil is one of the easiest ways to do this – will help with your baby's jaundice if you are breastfeeding as it will pass through your milk to your baby.

The sensitive newborn will also not be able to stay awake during motion until Weeks 8–12 onwards. Going out and about in the early days should therefore be restricted to nap times, I'm afraid, as your baby will most certainly fall straight to sleep when being cuddled in a sling or taken out in a car seat or pram. This in itself is restricting for you as a parent, I know, but by three months you will have a baby who sleeps beautifully at night, knows the difference between night and day and your day routine becomes non-restrictive – priceless! It's also important that your baby has enough still time to digest his milk before being put in a sling, pram or car seat and being moved around. Being taken out and jiggled around straight after a feed may make him vomit. Plan ahead for trips out: try to travel during nap times, feed your baby and give him awake time on arrival, and travel back during the next nap. Make sure all appointments are made over the nap time giving you enough time to feed and have awake time before having to wheel him out of the door.

As well as heat, light and motion, newborns are also very sensitive to noise. It's commonly thought by parents that being around chatter, the TV, music and background noises like the vacuum cleaner or washing machine will keep their little bundle awake. I'm afraid not ... in fact, quite the opposite. These background noises will lull your baby to sleep. Again, some babies are more sensitive to noise than others, but if your newborn falls asleep easily during feeds or awake time then make sure the only sounds he can hear are your voice and some stimulating toys. The Lamaze toys, like Jacques the Peacock, have stimulating hypnotic eyes, crinkle, rustle and squeaker sounds, as well as black-and-white patterns for fascinating visuals.

Interacting with your baby

At around Week 3 your newborn will start to wake up to the world and you may well be rewarded with the odd smile or two. Some newborns are free with their smiles, while others will be absorbing everything you do even if they don't seem to be responding for weeks and start to smile and coo at the same time. It's often thought that smiles this early are just down to wind, but it's easy to tell the difference. If your baby is focusing and reacting to your voice, face or pictures, it's a smile! Your baby will smile with his eyes and his whole face will light up, whereas a windy smile uses his mouth alone and usually his eyes will be closed. By encouraging stimulating play as early as one week old – as my routine does – you are engaging your baby's tiny brain and he will therefore react and start responding to stimulation much quicker than if you didn't.

At Weeks 6–8 your baby will start object tracking, following you around the room with his eyes and being able to track a mobile or moving picture. Toys and mobiles are for playtime only and should not be used to soothe your baby to sleep; they are stimulating for a newborn and therefore stop him from falling asleep. Mobiles should therefore be removed at bedtime. Although your baby can now see colour, pastel-coloured toys and mobiles are pretty useless at this early stage. Musical toys will also be of interest from Week 8, but be careful as if they are left on for too long they could lull your baby to sleep.

Unlike your baby's vision, his hearing is fully developed at birth. He will also love to hear you talking and singing, cooing, making exaggerated facial expressions, high-pitched noises and raspberry blowing. These noises will all be fascinating to him. Try sticking your tongue out and see if he copies you. Look at this time playing with your baby as another way to bond, instead of going straight in for a cuddle. When you are focusing on a routine which encourages structured awake time it's important that parents and visitors enjoy your baby in a way that enables him to stay awake when he is supposed to and not be sent to sleep by being cuddled by everyone.

As well as having one-on-one time with you, your baby needs time to play on his own. This builds his confidence and makes for a happy baby that you can put down to play while you are able to take care of yourself, making breakfast, expressing, organising siblings or simply going to the loo. The most obvious time for self-play is straight after your baby's day feeds, when he has a full tummy and has been close to you while being fed. Make use of this initial contented time. Towards the end of his playtime your baby will start to get grumpy and want to be entertained. In order to encourage your baby to increase his awake time, when he starts showing sleepy cues, you could distract him for an extra 10–15 minutes at a time until he reaches the full two-hour awake time at each feed period by Weeks 4–6. Overtiredness and sleeping cues are not an issue with newborns – this only becomes a problem with established babies from 3–4 months onwards.

Over the first 2–3 months, you may think that your baby's concentration will increase with age, but quite often it's the opposite. At around Weeks 6–8 your baby will become more aware of his surroundings, can see at a greater distance and will start to track and follow. He quickly becomes bored of static toys and pictures which have held his attention for a month or so and may become bored of being flat on his back on his play mat, only lasting 10–20 minutes at a time. Start using toy rotation to keep him entertained, by changing pictures and toys every 3–4 days, and move him to different play areas throughout the day: give him tummy time, use a baby chair instead of a play mat, have one-to-one chats with you or simply change rooms to play. You could also use mobiles, baby apps and musical toys before having a cuddle and quiet time and putting him down for a nap. This calm-down time is very important in order for your baby to settle to sleep. Allow 10–15 minutes of calming cuddling before bed.

Tummy time

Spending some time on his tummy is important for strengthening your baby's neck and developing his core strength. You can start 'tummy time' as soon as your baby is able to stay awake for over 1½ hours at any one feed period. Check your baby for wind first and leave at least half an hour after the feed for him to digest the milk before moving him on to his tummy, otherwise you can expect vomiting! Be aware: some babies like the tummy position so much that they fall asleep! If you don't start this early enough, some newborns will not like it but it's important to encourage tummy time on a daily basis as it develops your baby's core strength and lays the foundations to support his spine as an adult.

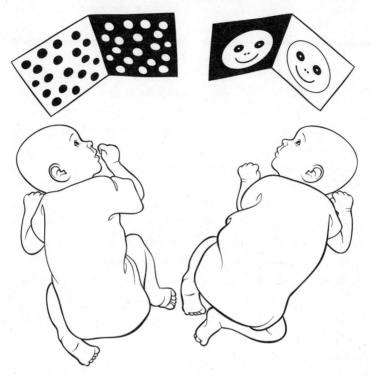

Stimulating tummy time

Awake time after feeds:
- Allows your baby to digest milk and relieve any excess wind. This is also the most content time of self-play, having a full tummy, clean nappy and being wind-free.
- Stimulates your baby's brain development.
- Builds confidence: your baby will be happy to play looking at black-and-white toys and taking in his surroundings without being held.
- Ensures better sleep at night and during daytime naps.
- Is a great way to bond and get to know each other, rather than simply cuddling. Your face is the best toy of all for your baby so one-to-one chats are a must.

In short ...

- Your baby's awake time can be gradually increased from 1–2 hours by Weeks 4–6, but please bear in mind that this is a guideline only and awake time will vary from baby to baby.
- Find a balance of both one-on-one playtime with you and some time for your baby to self-play on a play mat with black-and-white toys.
- Toys and mobiles will stimulate, not soothe, your baby and are for playtime only. Bedtime is for sleeping not playing.
- Allow a calm-down period of 10–15 minutes after play-time before your baby's naps and bedtime.
- Tummy time should be no less than 30 minutes after a feed to allow your baby digestion time. Tummy time helps develop your baby's core and neck muscles, which protect the spine.

Chapter Thirteen

Sleep, Settling and Sleep Positions

The 7pm to 7am Sleeping Baby Routine encourages good sleep patterns through progressively longer sleep at night and good-quality daytime naps. Teaching your baby the difference between night and day means a full night's sleep is reached much earlier than commonly thought. This should happen naturally as a result of your day routine. Sleeping through the night at an early age becomes part of your baby's routine and the earlier this is achieved the more habit-forming it becomes, so when hitting milestones such as teething your baby should be undisturbed by any discomfort. Encouraging a full night's sleep will form a solid sleeping habit which your baby will carry through toddlerhood, childhood and beyond. This is achieved by teaching positive associations with sleep and getting all the variables specific to your baby's needs correct, such as feeds, winding and structured awake time. When teaching your baby positive sleep habits, it makes sense that you create a good environment for your baby's sleep, encouraging naps and sleep in her cot or Moses basket with the odd pram or skin-on-skin nap. Napping on a play mat or in a baby chair will not encourage good, solid, quality sleep.

It's commonly thought that getting babies used to noise while sleeping means they will sleep anywhere without being woken. In the first few weeks this might be so, as your baby has not yet woken up to the world, but with a routine that achieves long periods of sleep at night so early on, it's unrealistic to think your baby would also have such deep sleep during the day, being able to sleep undisturbed by doors banging, other children running around, shouting or general day-to-day life going on. This is your trade-off – the longer a baby sleeps at night, the lighter and more easily woken she can be during the day until she has dropped one, or even two, of her daytime naps. Creating a good sleep environment ensures solid, undisturbed sleep. Sleep breeds sleep, so a baby who sleeps soundly during her daytime naps should also sleep soundly at night. Catnapping and frequently waking during the day has a knock-on effect on your nights.

Sleep aids

Babies are not born into the world needing to suck or be rocked to sleep. I believe one of the most important first steps of parenting is to teach your baby positive associations with settling. If a baby is well-fed and wind-free she should be able to settle to sleep without aid. Yes, you and your baby need lots of cuddle time, but if you cuddle your baby to sleep at each nap or through the night then that is how you are teaching her to sleep and at some point you are going to want to move on from this and have your baby sleep unaided. In my view, it is much easier and kinder to teach your baby positive sleep associations from the off. Make time for cuddles elsewhere during the day, such as before a nap, and maybe allocate one nap a day, or every other day, for a skin-on-skin nap with all your baby's other naps self-settled in her Moses basket, pram or cot.

The greater the settling task, such as endless pram pushing, rocking or using a dummy, the more you will need to do to help settle your baby as she gets older, making it increasingly hard to teach self-settling. The rocking gets lengthier, the need to wheel your baby out in the pram starts happening at every nap, and she becomes unable to sleep without motion. If you choose to use a dummy, eventually it will start falling out constantly, so you are up and down all night with frequent waking, with your baby needing yet more help to aid her back to sleep. Teaching positive associations with settling instils confidence in your baby to settle herself.

Lighting

For your baby's daytime naps, draw the curtains but do not fully black out the room; for night sleeping it should be totally blacked out. This is essential in the spring and summer months. Light flooding into the bedroom at 5am can interfere with sleep training. Blacking out the light at night teaches your baby the difference between night and day and also means less stimulation at night feeds or early morning waking when she is able to see more clearly and is aware of her surroundings (from around six weeks of age). Monitor lights, such as camera lights, can stimulate your baby if she wakes in the night and encourage waking. Use sticky black tape to cover any spotlights. This includes thermometer lights.

Lighting during the night feeds should also be kept to such a dim level that you can barely see to feed but instead have to feel your way around. This again avoids stimulation at night, which in turn helps your baby settle back to sleep.

Child night lights and musical toys are stimulating and will encourage waking and should not be used for newborns or babies.

Skin-on-skin naps

I encourage skin-on-skin naps once a day or at least once every other day, to enjoy and encourage emotional bonding. This also has the added benefit of increasing your milk supply. Prop yourself up slightly so your chest and head is at a 20–30° angle and tuck yourself into bed. Lay your baby on your chest (naked but with her nappy on) and enjoy a snooze together! Get prepared with everything you need around you as you will not be able to move for the duration of the nap. This also encourages you to nap which aids recovering. Skin-on-skin napping has a shelf life, and usually at around Weeks 6–8 a baby will find it hard to settle in that position, so make the most of it before this happens.

Of course, as per government guidelines around safe sleeping and reducing the risk of Sudden Infant Death Syndrome (SIDS), you should never share a bed with your baby if you have consumed alcohol, if you take drugs or if you're a smoker. It's also important never to sleep with your baby on a sofa or armchair.

Swaddling

Between three and six weeks the Moro (startle) reflex can really start kicking in, which means your baby is easily woken and may find it hard to settle as her arms and legs have no control, waving around, causing disruptive sleep. Swaddling is one of the best ways to keep your baby sleeping for longer. When they are swaddled, babies feel cuddled and secure while being able to sleep without being woken by the startle reflex.

Your newborn should learn to sleep with her arms free during the day – only introduce the day swaddle if her daytime naps are unsettled. Swaddling your baby for night sleeping only will help teach her the difference between night and day. Having said that, I would say that more than 75 per cent of the babies in my care need to be swaddled during the day due to the startle reflex. If you are starting my routine a little later on and are having problems with settling your baby for her daytime naps, then try swaddling during the day. I often hear parents commenting that their baby does not like being swaddled and prefers her arms out, but in my 20 years of sleep training, I've never known a baby not to like sleeping in a swaddle. They often don't like the process of being swaddled much, like a baby doesn't usually like being dressed, dried after a bath or even having her nappy changed, but a baby will sleep more peacefully in a swaddle.

When you use a swaddle, make sure it is made of thin, stretchy cotton (in my opinion, the Miracle Blanket®, made from a thin, stretchy cotton material, is the ideal swaddling blanket). Swaddle your baby across the chest and down around the body so no material is up around her face. The swaddle should be firmly fitted around her chest and arms, with her hips and legs fitted slightly looser. Please see the video on my website for how to safely swaddle your baby: www. thesleepingbabyroutine.co.uk.

The ideal sleeping environment is a room temperature of 18–21°C with your baby dressed in a vest bodysuit, a Babygro or sleepsuit, a swaddle, roll pillows (if using) and one thick, stretchy blanket or two thinner blankets to tuck her in. Do bear in mind that a baby's body temperature will vary, so if your room is 18°C and your baby's head feels cool, you will need to raise the temperature of the room slightly or add an extra blanket. It's important to find the right balance between keeping your baby warm and her not overheating.

Sleep Positions

Your baby's sleep position is so important. Having your baby sleep in a bouncy chair or on a play mat will not encourage good-quality sleep. Make sure you put your baby to sleep in her cot or Moses basket, or in the pram if you are going out (let her settle herself to sleep before pushing her out, thus allowing her to self-settle).

Current government advice is that your baby should sleep in a separate cot or Moses basket in the same room as you for the first six months, even during the day. However, I believe a baby needs her own space and environment to sleep well and to sleep undisturbed by parents moving around in the night and during the day. This also allows you to sleep more peacefully as newborns are mostly noisy little sleepers. If you are uncomfortable with this try putting your baby to sleep in her own room for daytime naps, but in the same room as you overnight. Try to give your baby her own space; respect her space and how easily she will be woken over the coming weeks. You will need to keep the room quiet and blacked out. Your baby will be going to bed at around 7.30pm – much earlier than yourself – so she may be disturbed as you go to bed. Another option is to put your baby in her own room for the first part of the night and move her once you have finished the first night feed. The government advice, which is based on theories, is, in my view, a precaution. I have been working with babies for 27 years and I have always put them to bed in their own, temperature-controlled, room.

I am very specific about sleep positions and the use of blankets, which should always be tucked in firmly, so there is no room for movement, and away from your baby's face. Camera monitors and breathing sensor pads are a popular way to keep an eye on your baby while she sleeps in her own room. The causes of SIDS are still unclear, but there is a lot of evidence that proves that environmental factors, such as smoking and overheating, and genetics contribute to the risks. Please do ensure you read the current advice and guidelines, and inform yourself about the causes of SIDS, before making a decision on where you put your baby to sleep. If you decide to follow my advice, it's important that you follow all the advice with regards to room temperature and blanket use.

In my experience, babies under 12 weeks of age sleep much better tilted slightly on their sides. However, the general advice given is to place babies to sleep on their backs and not on their sides, in case they roll on to their stomach. Using a roll pillow correctly stops this happening. The roll pillow also gives the added feeling of comfort on your baby's tummy and back, making her feel cuddled and secure. This sleep position also eliminates flat head syndrome – if you swap the side your baby is sleeping on every 24 hours, it makes for a perfectly round head. If you do choose to sleep your baby on her back and develop flat head syndrome it will, of course, resolve itself eventually, but it can cause neck movement restriction and tension.

Government guidelines advise back-sleeping only, which is blanket advice to stop parents sleeping their babies on their stomachs and to stop babies rolling on to their stomachs from their sides. As you can see in the image below, the baby's back is slightly tilted up and raised so she is not completely on her side but is tilted at a 30° angle. Before you make a decision on sleep positions, please check out current government guidelines, discuss side sleeping with a healthcare professional and watch the video on my website for how to use roll pillows safely: www.thesleepingbabyroutine.co.uk.

Roll pillows are best used in a Moses basket for ease as there is no movability. The roll pillow should only come up to chest height, as shown below, and have an even length roll on the front and back, which will enable you to tuck your baby in well. If you decide to follow my method then please make sure you use a roll pillow that is secure and is tucked in well.

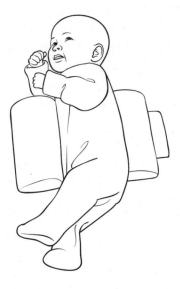

Sleep position using roll pillows advised on the 7pm to 7am
Sleeping Baby Routine

As the swaddling material and roll pillows can often raise your baby's body slightly higher than her head, always raise the head of the cot, pram or Moses basket slightly higher than the feet. Use a rolled-up muslin under the Moses basket mattress or a small blanket under the cot mattress to ever so slightly raise the angle. Of course, when raising the basket or cot make sure it is stable before putting your baby down to sleep. This should be a very slight raise so your baby's head is higher than her feet. If you raise it too high your baby may move down the mattress or to the side. Also ensure that you place your baby in the 'feet to foot' position, where her feet are at the end of the cot, Moses basket or pram. Please see my website for how to raise the cot safely: www.thesleepingbabyroutine.co.uk.

Tucking in

Tucking your baby into her cot, Moses basket or pram will make her feel secure and comforted, and also undisturbed by the Moro reflex, and she will be less likely to wake unnecessarily for the duration of her nap time. I help a lot of mothers remotely sleep train their babies and nine times out of ten they are not tucking their babies in. Tuck a blanket firmly into the basket, cot or pram at shoulder level to keep baby and blanket in place, and the blanket away from your baby's face.

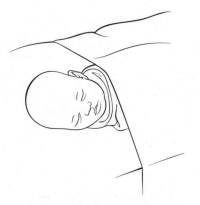

Sleeping baby tucked in securely

Please make sure there are no loose blankets! Not only is it dangerous for your baby as there is a danger of suffocation, but any loose blanket around your baby's face will encourage waking. The swaddle, roll pillows (if using) and tucked-in blanket will all help your baby sleep well and, once she is sleeping through the night, approaching four months and starting to move around in the cot, you can gradually take them away one at a time for a slow, smooth transition to sleeping in a sleeping bag.

A baby sleeping bag can be used once you are out of the newborn stage and your baby is able to roll around and move herself out of positions in her cot, from four months onwards. Start this process by moving your baby from her Moses basket to her cot once she is sleeping through the night for at least two weeks and has grown out of the basket. Do this during her daytime naps for a week or so before moving her over at night as well. Once your baby is sleeping through the night and if you are still swaddling her during the day, from 8–12 weeks, half swaddle your baby with one arm out, keeping the roll pillows (if using) and blankets firmly tucked in. If this is successful, take the swaddle away completely. If this is successful then do the same process at night, but keep the roll pillows (if using) and blankets until your baby starts moving in her cot. Only then take the roll pillows away. When blankets render useless, which is usually at around 5–6 months onwards, you should start using a sleeping bag and your baby is then free to sleep in any position in her cot. If any stage of this process is unsuccessful and your baby is unsettled and starts waking during the night or daytime naps, go back a step and try again in a week or so. Teaching your baby the difference between night and day and to sleep all night takes weeks, and sometimes months. Her sleep position, and keeping her tucked in and secure will help this process. Some babies love being tucked in to sleep and are reluctant to give up their newborn sleep position, while others will want the freedom and perhaps a free hand to chew on!

How to reduce the risk of SIDS

- Don't smoke during pregnancy or breastfeeding, and don't let anyone else smoke around your baby.
- Don't share a bed with your baby if you have consumed alcohol, if you take drugs or if you're a smoker.
- Don't sleep with your baby on a sofa or armchair.
- Don't let your baby overheat or get too cold.
- Keep your baby's head uncovered with blankets tucked in no higher than her shoulders.
- Place your baby in the 'feet to foot' position, with her feet at the end of the cot, pram or Moses basket.

Settling Techniques

Towards the end of your baby's awake/playtime and approaching her nap time, you will need to give your baby some 'you' time. In the first 6–8 weeks this can be more about stimulation as your baby increases her awake time, but gets bored on the play mat or various play stations. As your baby comes out of the newborn stage and is easily stimulated and aware of her surroundings, she will need calming and cuddling before bed. However, the idea is not to cuddle your baby to sleep, but to spend 10–15 minutes or so helping her to reach a comforted state and calm her active brain so she can settle herself. Don't expect your baby to be able to go straight from her play station to bed peacefully; she needs time to unwind before sleeping. I don't believe in newborns getting overtired, but I do believe in overstimulation.

When increasing your baby's awake time, this should be done gradually at the same time as her night sleeping gets more solid and longer. A newborn who needs to sleep will fall asleep anywhere and will not be woken if she indeed needs to sleep, so overtiredness is not a factor until she becomes interactive and aware of her surroundings at around Weeks 6–8. However, what can sometimes happen with newborns is, if she falls asleep before being put down for her nap and then wakes on being put down, it can be hard for her to resettle herself, and you may need to use the 'shush and hold' technique (see below).

Where possible, and I know this is tricky in the first four weeks, put your baby down to sleep while she is still awake or just about to drop off. Babies who fall asleep while being cuddled and then moved to their Moses basket or cot later, will often wake during transfer or simply because they are not where they fell asleep. Obviously putting your baby down awake is not always possible, as your newborn will often fall asleep before you have reached the Moses basket or cot, but as your newborn starts to become more aware it will become extremely important to encourage self-settling, so it is best to put it into practice as early as possible.

Always allow a few minutes for your baby to settle herself – she may look around and drift naturally or be quite vocal and have a bit of a yell before falling asleep. This is all normal as some babies are vocal in all they do. Use my two-minute rule (page 176) before going in and giving a helping hand with my 'shush and hold' technique. Shush and hold will only work if all the variables are met at each feed period: your baby is fed until she is full, is wind-free, has had enough awake time and has been tucked into her cot or Moses basket. The only time you would not wait for two minutes is after the bedtime feed. This is the only time of day your baby will go to bed on a full stomach. You may have missed a burp, which can cause discomfort or vomiting. This is your baby's biggest feed of the day and she needs to be wind-free to go to sleep on a full tummy.

Shush and hold

Before using my 'shush and hold' technique, wait for two minutes to see if your baby settles herself. If her crying is a stop–start intermittent cry, she may be half asleep and working out the settling process. The older your baby, the more stimulated she will be if you go in at this time and shush and hold may have the reverse effect and stimulate your baby awake. If she does not stop crying at whatever level is normal for her personally (some babies go straight to high-pitched screaming, while others sound more like they are shouting), you should go to assist and start with the shush and hold technique to help settle her.

Once you are sure that your baby needs some help to settle, put a hand on her body, press your cheek to her cheek and shush louder than your baby's cry. Babies respond to confidence and by raising your voice above your baby's cry, she will hear you, and by placing your hand and cheek on hers she will feel you and feel secure and reassured. As your baby's crying stops and her breathing calms, you will feel your baby relaxing. At this stage, quieten the shushing and slowly lift the pressure off, gently releasing your hand and cheek and quietly making your escape. Repeat the whole process again after waiting a further two minutes, if needed. If this doesn't work after the third attempt, swaddle your baby if she is not already swaddled and place her over your shoulder. Hold her firmly and pat her bottom while shushing and breathing deeply. Your breathing should calm and regulate your baby's breathing. If you are anxious and constantly changing her position and hold, jiggling and walking around feeling stressed and trying to calm her down, she will pick up on your anxiety and not feel secure. If you are relaxed and consistent in your method your baby will calm down. Again, once her breathing has calmed and relaxed, slowly stop shushing and gently put her down to bed. Tuck her in so she still feels some comforting pressure from the blanket. Cradling your baby in your arms is a feeding position and shouldn't be used for calming your baby – it quite often causes more upset and confusion. The most calming position is over your shoulder.

If the above settling technique doesn't work, check the following: did your baby feed well at her last feed; has she been winded well; and has she had enough awake time?

Twin Sleep Positions

Moses baskets are not needed with twins. They can sleep side-by-side at the foot of one cot to begin with. In the first four weeks lay them side-by-side without swaddles and without roll pillows during the day. Your babies will tend to mould into each other during the nap – so cute! It makes sense having grown together for almost nine months that they will sleep well being so close. At night, still sleep them side-by-side or either end at the foot of the cot, but swaddle your babies and use roll pillows if they fit and you choose to side-sleep your

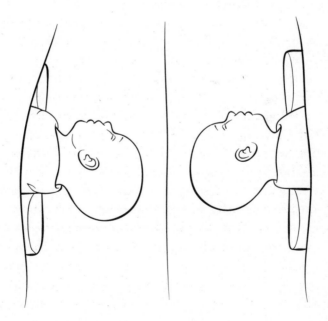

Twins positioned for sleeping at either end of a cot

babies, tucked in tight, as you would a single baby. Placing your babies so they face the same direction will cause less confusion as to which side they are sleeping on each night. Change direction every 24 hours. Laying them in the same order will cause less confusion to which baby is which at 3am! Using roll pillows side by side at night will stop your babies rolling into each other during the night. A baby needs her own personal space to release heat and keep her airways clear.

As your babies grow and need more room, or if they are waking each other up, they can then be separated. They can still sleep in the same cot, but instead sleep end-to-end. At around four months when they start to move in their cot or their heads are almost touching in the middle, move them to their own cots.

Chapter Fourteen

Troubleshooting

In the first three months of life your baby grows at the fastest rate, his digestive system is maturing, he becomes self-winding, he reaches his maximum intake of milk, and he becomes interactive and starts to communicate with you other than through crying. It's no wonder, then, that the routine can hit a few bumps along the way! During this stage you will no doubt face challenges and phases to overcome, such as wind and digestion, problems with settling, or bottle-feeding or milk flow issues, all of which may seem like a big deal at the time, but it's all a phase and you will soon move on to the next challenge. Welcome to parenting!

In this chapter I have outlined some common troubleshooting scenarios and questions to help you understand your new baby and iron out any bumps you may come across. I work with and help a lot of parents remotely, as well as hands-on, and come across a wide range of newborn-, baby- and child-related issues. Most of these issues can be resolved quickly by a process of elimination, which I constantly repeat and reiterate throughout this book. Newborns respond to their basic needs being met and if you are not meeting any one of them, your routine may not work. Babies who are already established and therefore in a routine of behaviour, even once their basic needs are met, may well have habitual behaviour with feeding and sleeping, especially if they have learned associations, such as being rocked or cuddled to sleep, sucking to sleep or snacking at feeds. Regardless of the baby's age, I ask my clients firstly to keep a diary to track their feed timings, milk intake, winding details, sleep positions and awake time so I can understand any patterns of behaviour that have been formed and then advise the following:

- Feed your baby until he is full at each day feed. Make sure your baby is actively sucking and not snoozing while feeding. Top up after the breast to make sure he is full. Increase your milk supply and express to understand your milk flow and what you are supplying.
- Gradually increase your baby's overall milk intake during the day.
- Wind your baby regularly – every 5–10 minutes on the breast or every 30ml (1oz) on the bottle, or whenever he is showing signs of comfort sucking and sleeping. Check for wind and burp your baby a few times after the feed during playtime while he is digesting his milk, usually 10–15 minutes apart.
- Encourage awake and playtime at each day feed, increasing the time your baby is awake to a full two hours at each feed period, which is usually easily reached by Weeks 4–6.

When troubleshooting and changing one aspect of your existing routine, such as alternative timings, a reduced pre-bath breast-feed or winding more frequently, allow at least three days for the technique to take effect before deciding to try another routine change. If you move on too quickly or try too many experiments at once, you won't know which part of the routine has worked and which part you still need to tweak to rectify your issue.

Feeding

My baby is really sleepy and falls asleep during feeding

Though a newborn baby – however she is being fed – will generally struggle to stay awake while feeding, this is often more of an issue with breastfed babies due to the comfort, body heat and closeness. The closeness of breastfeeding is a fantastic bonding experience but it often results in a baby sleeping more than feeding, which doesn't work well when establishing a routine. If you are bottle-feeding, try to find other times of day to cuddle and bond with your baby, such as having skin-on-skin naps together.

A newborn's body will heat up while feeding due to digestion, much as adults do when we eat, drink and digest food. Babies are extremely heat-sensitive, so creating the perfect environment to feed will help your baby to stay awake. Keep your baby cool by making sure the room temperature is between 19°C and 20°C for feeds. Regardless of her body temperature, your baby will still tend to comfort suck and drift off to sleep after a few minutes of suckling at the breast and will need to be winded every 5–10 minutes. On the bottle this would be after every 15–30ml (½–1oz). A newborn will not be able to actively feed for long periods. Active feeding and prompts, such as feet tickling while breast- and bottle-feeding, will help keep your baby focused. Stop regularly to keep your baby alert and also to wind her as sucking creates wind which can get trapped, swell in the stomach and give a false sense of fullness, which makes a newborn sleepy. If your baby starts to become inactive feeding and falls asleep, wake her by putting her down on a muslin on the floor and tickling her hands and feet until she is awake. Using a specific breastfeeding pillow, such as 'My Brest Friend', or a cushion to bottle-feed will help to keep your baby awake as well as ensuring a good feeding posture.

Wake your baby 10–15 minutes before each day feed to ensure she is ready and enthusiastic for the feed. Do this by stripping off her clothes so she is down to her vest bodysuit and her arms and legs are exposed. Though your baby's hands and feet may feel cool, her body should still be warm and this is where you should feel to check her body temperature. Your baby will need to be wide awake for her feed and not have spent the whole 15 minutes waking up. If she wakes and cries straight away, try to distract her or walk her around over your shoulder without sending her back to sleep. A baby going straight on the breast from sleep will no doubt fall straight back to sleep after a few sucks. Make sure there is no background noise, such as too much chatter, the TV or household appliances. Move to a quieter, cooler room to focus on feeding if necessary.

It's normal for babies to fall asleep after a feed, but this is a result of a full tummy and digestion, not being tired. Waking your baby with a tepid to cool water nappy change will help wake and revive her for awake time, which is essential for digestion during the day. Not encouraging enough awake time after feeds and letting your baby catnap will lead to a habit of catnapping and not being able to have solid time awake or asleep, which will result in frequent waking during the day and night and an inability to stay awake for her feeds. Even if your baby's awake time is as little as 15–20 minutes, you can gradually increase the time as she grows. This ensures your baby is sleeping for the right reason and not due to digestion.

Babies born in the summer months can be especially hard to wake during the day. Heat and humidity can cause havoc with a routine. Strip washes and a slightly cooler bath than her normal bath temperature (30–32°C rather than 34–35°C) will help cool and revive her before, during or after a feed.

In the first 3–4 weeks of life, a baby's waking time may vary and it is, of course, more important to stay awake while being fed than it is having two hours' awake time to include the playtime. Your baby's awake time will need to build as she grows, until she is established and out of the newborn phase. With some babies, no two days will be the same so be prepared to be flexible.

It's also important to note that most newborns will feed with their eyes shut, so try to focus on your baby's feeding activity. If she is actively sucking and swallowing with her eyes shut, she is awake; if she starts to comfort suck and therefore feeding becomes inactive and her eyes are closed, she will inevitably fall asleep. The idea is to stop this happening.

My baby is falling asleep during the bedtime bottle

Firstly make sure your bedtime routine is tight timewise:

- Awake at 5.45pm
- Pre-bath feed at 6pm
- Bath at 6.30pm
- Post-bath bottle at 6.45pm

This should leave you with 45–60 minutes for the post-bath bottle.

It's natural for babies to fall asleep at this time of day and is actually something you want them to do moving forward – this is bedtime after all. It's the only time of day your baby will have the bulk of her feed at the end of her awake time and before bed. Treat this feed like any other day feed – keep your baby awake by keeping her cool, ensure she is actively feeding and wind her every 15–30ml (½–1oz). Give the bottle-feed in the room in which she sleeps, away from noisy siblings or background noises such as the TV or household appliances. Background noise will send a baby to sleep during the establishing newborn phase.

Make sure the bath temperature is no more than 34–35°C. This may feel cool to you, but it will be warm to a baby who is heat-sensitive. A bath that is too warm for even a short amount of time – as little as five minutes – has the same relaxing effect of a 20-minute, warm/hot bath for an adult. If the water is too warm, the effects of the bath will mean your baby will start to fall asleep on the bottle before she has taken enough milk.

Make sure your baby is not having too much milk before her bath. If you are breastfeeding, by Week 4 your milk flow will speed up as your milk thins. Reduce the amount of time your baby feeds on the breast by five minutes each side and see if this helps with her enthusiasm for the bottle. Give no more than 60ml (2oz) at the pre-bath feed if you are bottle-feeding.

If you are still having problems keeping your newborn awake for the bedtime bottle, try my temporary trick of a 45-minute bed break. This works short-term but should not be kept as part of your regular routine in the long-term. I use this trick when a baby is unable to stay awake and unable to take the milk she regularly takes to set her up for the night. Have a cut-off point from feeding, waking and winding at 7.30/8pm. Put your baby to bed as you would for the night, swaddled and tucked in. Wake her back up 45 minutes later which allows her stomach to digest the last feed a little and enough time asleep in order to be woken briefly for a few more ounces. A 30-minute bed break is too short and your baby will be hard to wake up, while an hour could be too long and she may decide that she is ready for another awake cycle. Your baby may, of course, once put down to bed for the 45-minute bed break, decide she is actually hungry and be ready to feed within minutes of putting her down. If this is the case, get her back up, un-swaddle her and offer more milk. Do not rely on this break to give any more milk than a 30–60ml (1–2oz) booster feed as you must focus on giving your baby the majority of her milk after the bath and during the time allocated for this bottle.

While this is a trick I have frequently used over the last 20 years, I have never known a baby be able to wake back up and take more than 60ml (2oz) if the routine is being followed properly and she has fed well during the day. Before offering more milk, change your baby's nappy to help revive her, and check for wind that has formed while digesting.

Can I delay this 45-minute bed break and introduce a dream feed so my baby takes more milk?

You can, but then you won't have the benefit of my routine helping you and your baby sleep through the night as quickly as you may have liked. My routine encourages solid sleep with night waking gradually getting later through the night as your day routine starts to take effect, with the majority of milk intake and awake time happening during the day. The staggered feed at bedtime allows your baby to have her largest feed at this time and, if woken for a dream feed at around 10–11pm, she should be disinterested in milk. Dream feeds do work if you are not doing the staggered feed, but they encourage feeding at night and therefore have a knock-on effect on all your day feeds. The more milk your baby is given at night, the less she will take during the day. This also means that you stay up to feed and get to bed much later and effectively only get half a night's sleep. The dream feed method is often a longer process of helping your baby to sleep through the night.

I am doing a dream feed with my baby and want to drop it

Firstly introduce the staggered feed as part of your new routine, giving as much milk as your baby naturally takes after the bath. You then have two options: stop waking your baby at night for the dream feed and see when she naturally wakes for a feed, giving no more than a 120ml (4oz) bottle or 20–30 minutes on the breast, including winding. Alternatively, you can change the time of the dream feed, nightly, until it is phased out. Waking your newborn earlier for a feed will help to stop habitual waking for the dream feed. Gradually reduce the amount of milk given for the dream feed or limit it to 120ml (4oz), depending on how much milk your baby is used to having at this time. If she is used to having 240ml (8oz), you might find that 120ml (4oz) is not enough to settle her back to sleep. If she is having 150–180ml (5–6oz) then 120ml (4oz) should be enough to settle her. If breastfeeding for the dream feed, reduce the time on each breast by 5–10 minutes nightly until phased out. As the quantity of milk at the dream feed is reduced, look to increase the post-bath feed and your baby's overall daily milk intake to compensate for the loss of milk at the dream feed as it is phased out.

I am having trouble increasing my baby's milk intake at the bedtime bottle

The bedtime bottle should increase to 150–240ml (5–8oz) by Weeks 6–8. This bottle is increased gradually, 15–30ml (½–1oz) maximum at a time, which is a very gentle increase. The last 30ml (1oz), and even the last five minutes of any breast- or bottle-feed, will always be slow, and it will sometimes be hard to keep your baby awake or interested as she becomes full. Your baby is growing fast, and so is her appetite, but she may not recognise this as the most important feed of the day. That and your baby naturally being tired at this time of day can make this milk increase tricky. If you are having trouble increasing this bottle-feed, here are a few things to check.

Your baby's pre-bath milk intake should be no more than 60ml (2oz) from a bottle, only increasing to 90ml (3oz) once she is taking over 240ml (8oz) post-bath. Pre-bath breastfeeding should be capped at a maximum of 15 minutes on each breast. If you have fast-flowing milk your baby could be getting way too much milk at this time and therefore affecting her milk intake after the bath. Some mothers whose milk literally flows out in one go will need to reduce this feed down to as little as five minutes each side, or give one breast for 5–10 minutes only and then express the other breast. This avoids giving your baby too much milk and two lots of foremilk. Your milk supply depletes throughout the day and will eventually fall short of your baby's demand, but you may still provide more than enough milk for the pre-bath feed. Reduce this feed by five minutes each breast at a time until your post-bath issues are resolved.

Slow the pre-bath feed down with more winding breaks so as to not finish the feed too quickly. If your baby feeds too fast, she may not realise she has eaten and be unhappy when you restrict this feed. Newborns are born with the fight-or-flight instinct and will generally cry until they are fed or the edge has been taken off their hunger. If you have reduced this pre-bath feed to 5–10 minutes, slow it down with two-minute winding intervals, which will lengthen the feed and give her enough time to tell her brain she has eaten. As your baby grows and becomes aware of her surroundings, this short feed will no longer be an issue as she gets used to this restricted feed being part of her routine. Regardless of the length of the pre-bath feed, keep bath time at 6.30pm. This feed and bath period is your baby's fourth awake period of the day and is spaced out to allow enough awake time before bed.

Make sure your baby's afternoon and evening feeds are at least 3½ hours apart, increasing to four-hourly if the pre-bath feed advice on shortening the feed doesn't apply to you. Change your 2.30pm feed to 2pm and adjust the other day feeds accordingly. Increasing the time between these two feeds allows a greater increase in appetite. The downside is that the afternoon nap is the first to become unsettled and dropped completely so increasing the distance between the two feeds will not work if your baby doesn't get enough sleep in the afternoon as she will be too tired for the bottle, let alone trying to increase her milk intake.

If your baby is unsettled and does not sleep well in the afternoon, try extending her awake time to 2¼ hours after the 2pm feed, which will help to encourage a longer afternoon nap.

Make sure the bath temperature is not too warm, which can make newborns sleepy after the bath. The ideal bath temperature is 34–35°C.

Wind your baby thoroughly even if she is only having 60ml (2oz) pre-bath. If breastfeeding and capping the time on the breast to, say, 8–10 minutes, break to wind every two minutes and make sure you are following a wind-free diet so you are not adding fuel to the fire and creating more wind which fills your baby's tummy instead of milk (see page 34). This will upset your baby's milk intake on the bedtime bottle and could cause vomiting due to trapped wind which builds up during the day. Also wind your baby after the bath and before the bottle as even a little amount of milk pre-bath will create wind while she is digesting, especially after sloshing around in the bath. Nine times out of ten, I will get a burp up while baby is still wrapped in her towel and is over my shoulder walking from the bath to the changing table.

During the post-bath bottle, break to wind your baby every 30ml (1oz), and even at 15ml (½oz) intervals for the last 60ml (2oz). The greater the milk intake the more wind created while sucking and digesting. Less trapped air = greater milk intake.

My baby looks very hungry at the pre-bath feed and would easily take more milk. Why do you not advise giving more than a 30-minute breastfeed or a 60ml (2oz) bottle?

This pre-bath feed is to make the bath time calm and take the edge off your baby's hunger. Giving more milk at this time increases the risk of vomiting on the post-bath bottle, as your baby will have been sloshed around in the bath. It will also interfere with your baby's appetite after the bath. The idea is to increase your baby's post-bath milk intake until it is the biggest feed of the day, taking enough milk to set her up for a full night's sleep.

Wouldn't feeding longer on the breast or giving more than 120ml (4oz) in the middle of the night help my baby sleep for longer?

Yes, but only temporarily as you will be encouraging heavier feeds at night which will encourage night waking in the long-term. My routine is a plan to help your baby sleep through the night and to do this you need to cap the night feeds in order to increase your baby's milk intake during the day. The more milk given at night the harder it is to increase the day feeds, and so it goes on. Say you have six feeds a day, making an overall intake of 720ml (25oz). If two of these are night feeds, then 240ml (8oz) of the total daily intake will be given at night. Increasing each of these two feeds by just 30ml (1oz) at each night feed would mean that your night feeds would be bigger than those in the day. Night feeds should give your baby just enough milk to settle her, not to fill her up. The day feeds should be your focus and, as these increase, your baby's appetite will decrease at night and night feeds will eventually phase out as she takes the majority of her milk during the day. You must, however, give your baby enough milk at the night feeds (120ml/4oz) for her to be able to settle for four hours or more. Giving too little during the night may result in frequent waking.

Babies tend to be more efficient at night if they have woken themselves to feed. If you are up to feed in the night, invest in this feed by giving the right amount of milk for the time of night and wind your baby properly:

- 11pm–3am: 30 minutes maximum or 120ml (4oz) bottle
- 3am–4am: 20 minutes maximum or 90–100ml (3–3½oz) bottle
- 4am–5am: 10–15 minutes maximum or 60–90ml (2–3oz) bottle
- 5am–6am: No feed zone, cuddle back to sleep

(These timings include winding.)

Why can I not give the other breast after the bath as I have milk left over?

While you may currently have more than enough milk for the pre-bath feed, you may not have enough milk for the total combined feed and, certainly by Weeks 6–10, you will not have enough milk to meet your baby's demand for her biggest feed to see her through the night. If you don't encourage the bottle in the early weeks as part of the routine now, she may reject the bottle and fall asleep on the breast after the bath having not taken enough milk, due to the soporific effects of breastfeeding and naturally being tired. As a result, your baby will not sleep as long as you might like or through the night.

The bedtime bottle is key to the success of your routine moving forward. During this establishing stage your baby will learn that the bottle is part of her routine and it will help her to recognise that bedtime is coming. Giving breast milk or formula in a bottle at this time of day is more efficient as your baby is less likely to fall asleep and you are aware of how much milk she is drinking. Any breast milk expressed and not used during your 24-hour period can be frozen (for up to six months) and saved for weaning or if you ever need to supplement.

Friends are waking their babies up at 10pm or 11pm for a dream feed. Why do you not advise this?

I don't believe in waking babies and encouraging heavy feeds during the night. Instead, I give a much larger feed before bed with the staggered feed. This and the effects of the routine ensure your baby has enough milk to sleep for 4–6 hours during the first part of the night. The length of sleep will naturally increase until she eventually sleeps through the night. With the staggered feed before bed she will not be hungry for a feed at 10–11pm so if you implement a dream feed you would be encouraging a feed she has not naturally woken for or needs. Another reason not to wake your baby for a feed at this time is that you'll probably wait up for the feed and not get to bed until, perhaps, midnight. During the newborn stage and while feeding at night you should ideally be going to bed early, at around 9–10pm at the latest, not halfway through the night. You need sleep to maintain a good milk supply and for your body to recover from the birth. The staggered feed technique means your baby sleeps undisturbed at night and naturally wakes when she needs to feed. This method helps babies sleep longer at night, and through the night, quicker than a baby on the dream feed method.

I am finding it very difficult to wind my newborn

Firstly, your newborn needs to be awake in order to wind her effectively – you can't wind a sleeping baby. Babies fall asleep constantly while feeding, so make sure you have the perfect feeding environment – a quiet, cool room so your baby can focus on feeding.

Wind increases with the increase of milk intake, making new-borns generally harder to wind/burp at around Weeks 4–6, when their milk intake more than doubles. A baby will need to burp every 30ml (1oz) or 5–10 minutes on the breast until her digestive system strengthens and she begins to self-wind at around Weeks 8–12. Winding a baby should only take a few minutes. Do not spend 10 minutes winding as you will be cutting into her feeding time. At the beginning of the feed, if you are struggling to get a burp out, simply give a little more milk and try again, after 15ml (½oz) or 2–3 minutes on the breast. If you are halfway through the feed and your baby is obviously drinking at the breast or has taken at least 30ml (1oz) you will need to work harder to get the burp out. Try different winding positions (see page 9). Lay your baby on a muslin on the floor, flat on her back, and push her knees into her tummy and chest firmly and then stretch her legs back out straight. I like to do this three times before lifting her up and letting her body stretch out briefly before placing her back on my knee to wind again. This will help encourage the air to come up. If your baby is prone to vomiting easily then don't use this technique at the end of the feed and when using this technique do not leave her there for more than a minute or two. I stay clear of the winding position that lies a baby face down across your knees. On my routine you are feeding your baby meals and an upside-down baby will more than likely be sick.

Sometimes too much winding can hold air bubbles down instead of pushing them up and can also send your baby to sleep. If your baby is sleepy do not wind her over your shoulder. When your usual winding technique doesn't work, try a gentler approach with a little tummy pressure and tickle her sides. Sit her on your knee as if she is sat on a chair with her legs dangling over your knee, head held up straight and in line, supporting her with a little pressure on her tummy. The stomach muscles have not yet developed and she is unable to use them to support herself until she is around 8–10 weeks old. You will need to hold your baby's diaphragm up. Tickle gently around her sides to coax the wind out. As your baby grows you will be able to feel where the wind is and focus on that area to help push the air up and out.

If you are breastfeeding and your baby is comfort sucking or you have run out of milk you will not get a burp out. Your baby needs to be actively drinking milk for the need to be winded.

If you are bottle-feeding, get the perfect shape teat and bottle for your baby's mouth and suck. The teat should be size one for the first 8–12 weeks and must fit well in your baby's mouth. Too fast or too slow sucking can make for a windier baby. Generally the more awake your baby is and the more active the sucking and feeding, the easier a baby is to wind and the more air is released.

My 10-week-old baby wants to chat instead of feed, which is lovely, but how do I get her to feed?

From around six weeks of age, babies become interactive and start smiling and cooing. This is beautiful and often brings a tear of joy to my eye ... but it often disrupts feeds which have just started being super-efficient as your baby is now able to stay awake for the whole feed period. Once the edge has been taken off her hunger, your baby may decide that it's time to play, smile and chat instead of continuing to feed after the first breast or a few ounces on the bottle. This results in lower milk intake during the day which can have an impact on your nights or mean your baby has not had enough milk to sustain her until the next feed time. In the early days, waking your baby 10–15 minutes before a feed was to make sure she was fully awake and ready to feed. Now this 10–15 minutes should be used for 'chat' time. Use this time to really engage with your baby, chat to her and say your hellos before feeding, which will allow your baby to focus on the feed. Try not to chat during feeds and when breaking to wind to help keep the feed focused.

If this doesn't work, give your baby a five-minute break – wind her, change her nappy, have a little chat, and then continue the feed – but try to keep the feed as close to an hour as possible, otherwise you will be encouraging snacking.

You may find your baby is now easily distracted when feeding. Feeding in company with siblings or with the TV on can cause stop–start feeding. Try to create a calm, quiet environment to combat this.

My baby screams when first latching on to the breast. Could it be the speed of my milk flow?

Babies are born with a fight-or-flight instinct when they are hungry and will usually cry until they are fed. For some babies this can sound quite dramatic and they will not calm down until they have taken enough milk to take the edge off their immediate hunger. If your breasts have a slight delay on the let-down of milk this can frustrate a newborn. A delayed let-down can mean that your baby sucks and falls off crying until the milk is released. To combat this you can hand express for a few minutes before latching your baby on or use a breast pump for 30 seconds to encourage your milk flow.

Too quick a let-down may flood your baby with milk when they are at their most enthusiastic point of feeding. This can cause great discomfort with wind and frustration, and can mean they come off the breast crying. To combat this issue, express 30ml (1oz) from each side before latching your baby on, taking off some of the foremilk which will slightly slow the speed of your milk flow. With fast-flowing milk you will need to wind your baby more frequently. Instead of the usual 5–10 minutes, try winding your baby at two-minute intervals, 2–3 times, and then extend this to four minutes, six minutes, and so on. This more frequent winding is to accommodate your baby's quick milk intake. If you don't wind more frequently with a fast milk flow, the milk speed and greater milk intake can cause trapped wind and vomiting due to your baby having taken in too much milk too quickly. The upside is that by 6–8 weeks your day feeds could take as little as 30 minutes and night feeds 10–15 minutes in total. With fast-flowing breast milk you will need to decrease the pre-bath feed to 5–10 minutes each side or 10 minutes on one side only and express the other side.

My newborn screams and pushes my breast away at the start of a feed

Babies with the fight-or-flight instinct can be like crazed little fluffy animals until milk hits their tummies and the edge is taken off their hunger. They may look like they are pushing away but they are often trying to do the opposite and latch on to the breast, but are getting frustrated and frantic until they are able to. A baby who has latched on well for weeks may hit a growth spurt and, in her new-found urgency to feed, will not be able to latch on to the breast and get upset. Babies have no control over their hands during the newborn stage and are unable to push your breast away, even if it looks like they are physically doing so. Calm your baby over your shoulder, shush her gently and then try again.

It's also important to check your baby's feeding position and try latching her with a different position, such as the rugby/football hold (see page 41). She may find it easier to latch on to the other breast and it might be worth starting on that side after a few unsuccessful attempts to latch on to the first breast. Always attempt to alternate your starting breast otherwise you may become uneven and produce more milk on the favoured side. Make sure your baby's head and body are properly supported while feeding.

Your baby's behaviour could also be down to the speed of the milk flow as foremilk sprays too fast into her mouth. If this is the case, it will be more apparent during the morning feed when your milk supply is at its greatest. Try expressing the first 30ml (1oz) off each side before latching your baby on.

If you are mixed feeding and have a low milk supply, you could have a case of breast rejection, though this is extremely rare. This shouldn't interfere with latching on, but when your baby starts to suck and is not rewarded with milk she will become upset, bob on and off the breast, cry or just fall asleep while comfort sucking, only to go through it all again every time you latch her on or break to wind. Your baby will still be hungry and her appetite is not being satisfied. This makes the issue a milk supply issue, not a rejection issue. Check this by expressing straight after the feed to see if there is any milk left. Could your breasts have run out of milk? See page 29 for advice on increasing your milk supply.

Tongue tie can also cause latching problems and therefore frustration and distress. A baby with tongue tie is unable to hold her latch as her tongue cannot stay forward to suck. Ask your midwife to check your baby and if there is even a minor tongue tie and you are having latch problems then get your baby's tongue tie snipped. This should sort your baby's latch and her sucking issues. Cutting a tongue is a simple snip of skin which causes brief discomfort, only to be forgotten about quickly when sucking.

A high palate (which is often misdiagnosed as tongue tie) and a recessed lower jaw can also cause problems with latching. Try and make sure your nipple goes up into the roof of your baby's mouth and seek advice from your midwife or health visitor with latching. It's common for babies to be born with a recessed jaw and chin and for it to move into the correct position within a few days after birth.

My baby keeps rejecting the bottle

Sometimes introducing a bottle can be tricky. If you are breastfeeding and only giving your baby one bottle a day at the bedtime feed, it's natural for her to prefer the breast. That's one of the reasons I introduce the bottle in the first two weeks of life. The later you introduce a bottle the more chance there is of bottle rejection. Even if you do follow my routine from the start you can come up against bottle rejection as the weeks go on. This is usually around Weeks 5–8 when your baby becomes more aware. The time of day you are giving the bottle is when your baby will be at her most tired and irritable. The rejection may not be due to the bottle as such, but the fact that the breast is more comforting. As your milk supply depletes during the day, the bedtime bottle is key to helping your baby sleep through the night so early on.

To test if your baby really is rejecting the bottle, offer her a bottle at the mid-morning feed and express instead of breast-feeding. If she takes the bottle without a problem, it's the time of day that's an issue so you might need to start the bedtime feed a bit earlier, but don't miss out the pre-bath feed and bath. Try reducing the pre-bath breastfeed by five minutes each side at a time and see if that makes a difference to her enthusiasm for the bottle, as you might be giving too much milk pre-bath. You could also temporarily swap the pre-bath breastfeed for a 60ml (2oz) bottle and see if the post-bath bottle improves. If your baby refuses the bottle at the mid-morning feed but takes the breast without a problem then you most certainly have bottle rejection. Make sure you are using the correct shape and size teat (see page 102 for more advice on this).

Most babies will get used to the bottle if you are consistent with it. You could add an extra bottle-feed during the day for a week and express that feed instead, to encourage bottle-feeding and, once you are over the bottle issue, change that feed back to the breast. Do this during the day and not for night feeds. You want your night feeds to remain light on milk, quick, easy and comforting.

If you have started with the bottle from the beginning, have bottle-fed with no issues and suddenly come up against bottle rejection, do persevere and be consistent with the routine and it will eventually click back into place. Be assured that this is just a phase and, as I said before, it can take the whole of the newborn stage to become established with feeding and sleeping. Who gives this bottle can make all the difference to its success. Often dads coming home from work to do the bath and bedtime bottle can suddenly come up against bottle rejection. This happens when your baby becomes more aware and, having had Mum breastfeeding all day, suddenly doesn't want Dad to feed. Your baby could also reject the bottle from Mum and only take it from Dad because she is used to being fed from the breast by Mum. This bottle rejection is not due to 'smelling' your milk, but your baby being aware of how you feed and, of course, she does not associate Dad with breast-feeding. Again this phase will pass. Create a calm environment to feed and pass the feeding baton back to Mum or Dad for a few weeks if necessary.

Another time babies suddenly start to reject their bottle is at around four months when their rate of growth slows and they tend to go off their milk and start teething. Early weaning would be a good option here to take the pressure off your baby's milk intake. I advise to start weaning from four months if needed and your baby is ready to be weaned. You can then take the process extremely slowly and without pressure. I introduce solid food in the morning to allow the stomach to digest and not interfere with your nights.

If you are introducing the bottle from Week 4 onwards and starting the routine at a later stage, bottle rejection could be an issue that you are unable to resolve. I have a few tricks you could try to encourage your baby to take the bottle:

- giving a 60ml (2oz) bottle pre-bath and saving the breast milk supply for after the bath;
- putting your baby to bed on bottle refusal and waking her up for a feed after a 45-minute bed break;
- offering a bottle before the breast during the day to increase her overall milk intake, so she gets used to the bottle and realises the bottle is her friend.

It is very rare, but I have known a few babies who have out-right refused to take the bottle and screamed at every attempt at giving it to them, no matter what time of day, teat shape or tricks I have used to encourage them. When this does happen you will need to change the routine which will no doubt inter-fere with your quest for a full night's sleep. Increase your milk supply as much as you can and make sure you have a rich diet so your breast milk is nutritionally dense and filling. Give a 15–20-minute maximum breastfeed pre-bath on one side. The faster the flow of milk the less you should offer at this time, saving the majority of your supply for the post-bath feed.

It's worth trying the bottle every so often or weekly to see if your baby changes her mind. Speak to a health visitor about starting weaning at four months to increase your baby's daily food intake and therefore her likelihood of sleeping through the night.

My newborn is still hungry after a breastfeed

It sounds like your milk supply is not meeting your baby's demand. Look to increase your milk supply, expressing after feeds to check if you have any milk remaining and to stimu-late supply. Top your baby up after a 50-minute breastfeed with a 30–60ml (1–2oz) bottle to start with. If this goes down easily then increase it to 90ml (3oz). Your supply will deplete throughout the day so your top-ups will need to increase as the day goes on.

Make sure your baby is actively sucking at the breast and not drifting off to sleep. An active suck will be a wide circular action and you should be able to see a swallow and sometimes hear your baby drinking. Comfort sucking, and therefore not drinking or stimulating your breast, looks like a short up-and-down action with a pause, nibble-nibble, stop, munch-munch, pause. Your baby is unlikely to be getting any milk with this action so break to wake and wind her. When you re-latch with a more enthusiastic baby, massage and squeeze down through the breast to help her extract any remaining milk. Teamwork is key when you are trying to get your baby to drain your breast.

I struggle to wake my baby for her feeds

Most newborns fall asleep when feeding, especially on the breast. I am forever de-latching and waking babies up to re-latch them back on to the breast to encourage active sucking until they get into the swing of things and are able to stay awake by themselves by Weeks 6–10. Wake your baby up at least 10–15 minutes before her feed and take off her clothes down to her vest bodysuit. Check the room is not too warm (it should be around 19–20°C). Put her on her play mat or a muslin on the floor (not a warm, comfy Moses basket or over your shoulder!), tickle her hands and feet and try a cool water nappy change to stimulate her awake. You may feel bad about waking your baby for feeds during the day – as the saying goes 'Let sleeping babies lie' – but if you don't wake her she will inevitably wake you more often at night as she has a reduced milk intake during the day. Once her eyes are open and she is looking around, make eye contact to stimulate her and check that she is fully awake. If she is not properly awake, she will just fall asleep again within minutes of starting the feed. Keep up the stimulation for 10 minutes until she is ready to feed.

Try hard not to let her fall asleep while feeding as she will be much harder to wake back up once she has actually fallen asleep and taken the edge off her hunger. Whenever she shows signs of dropping off to sleep, stop feeding, sit her up and tickle her hands and feet or put her back on her play mat before winding. Falling asleep during the feed can be a particular problem with the bedtime feed – this is hardly surprising as it is nearly bedtime. Newborns will most likely spend most of their time sucking with their eyes closed; this doesn't mean they are asleep. If your baby is actively sucking and swallowing she is awake, but once she starts to comfort suck and use your breast for comfort, much like a dummy, she will soon drift off to sleep. The idea is to prevent comfort sucking which leads to dozing.

Changing the routine slightly will make it easier to wake your baby successfully for feeds. You could temporarily change your feeding routine to four-hourly which will allow a greater build-up of appetite and also allow more time for naps between feeds, which should ensure more enthusiasm and wakefulness. The only issue with feeding four-hourly is that there is no flexibility with the feeding times. Another option would be to limit playtime: shorten one or each awake period to 1½ hours to ensure each nap period is two hours, encouraging more sleep than awake time. If naps become unsettled as a result then you will need to extend the awake time back to two hours.

Option three is to wake your baby 20 minutes before the feed giving a longer awake time. Newborns will take longer to wake from a skin-on-skin nap or being pushed in the pram. They will also find it hard to wake if there is too much noise, heat or light.

I don't feel I am producing enough milk

It is quite normal for mothers to take up to six weeks to establish a good milk supply. Supply and demand means supply comes after your baby's demand. Your body is recovering from giving birth and is using energy to do so. The more rest your body has to recover the more milk you will supply. The more active stimulation your baby gives your breast at each feed the more milk you will supply. Eating well, drinking lots of water and fennel tea, destressing and relaxation also play a big role in milk production. Expressing after each day feed will not only increase your supply but will help you understand how much milk you are producing. As well as keeping a baby diary, keep an expressing diary so you can keep track of your milk supply. Try and express at the same times after a feed and at the same time in the evening once your baby is waking after 12am. You should gradually see an increase in milk and be able to work out if and why you see a decrease in your milk supply, which could be due to being tired or not drinking enough that day. Maybe you see an increase after having a skin- on-skin nap with your baby. Massaging your breast at the end of each breastfeed and while expressing will help to drain your breast and you can see which areas to apply pressure to to help reach the last of the hindmilk.

It's not the end of the world if you have to give the occasional top-up bottle after a breastfeed until your supply increases. For some mothers this is the only way to get more sleep at night. The top-up milk will fill your baby up during the day which will ensure she sleeps well at night, letting you sleep well which results in an increased milk supply. Having to get up and feed every two hours at night means you will be sleep-deprived which will leave you with a lower milk supply. See page 29 for more advice on increasing your milk supply.

If I offer a bottle will my baby reject the breast?

No! I have never had a baby reject the breast as a result of offering a bottle. The one bottle a day, as advised on my routine, will not interfere with breastfeeding. What can happen, if you are mixed feeding and you are not encouraging active sucking while breastfeeding and do not have a good milk supply, is that a baby can become lazy on the breast as the bottle is easier to drink from. Also, if you don't stimulate your breast and offer every feed as a breastfeed in the first two weeks, most babies will find the bottle easier and prefer the bottle. A bottle top-up should be just that – a top-up – and not the majority of your baby's milk intake. If your baby is breastfeeding and actively sucking, latching on well and enjoying her feeds, introducing a bottle before bed and a few top-ups during the day if needed will not result in breast rejection. Babies simply prefer the breast to a bottle.

On the other hand, not introducing a bottle early on could cause you problems later when you need to wean your baby from breast to bottle (for example, if you go back to work or just want to go out for an evening). She is more likely to reject the bottle if it is sprung on her weeks down the line.

My midwife/NCT counsellor/best friend says that if I top up with formula I'll start to produce less milk and end up having to stop breastfeeding. Is this true?

No, not unless you are replacing breastfeeds with formula. Skipping breastfeeds, even in the night, will reduce your milk supply. When your baby naturally sleeps later through the night you will be expressing before bed and so adding extra stimulation. Eventually your breasts will get into a routine and manage to supply all the milk needed during the day but while your baby is waking at night, you should breastfeed and not skip the feed. Giving your baby a bottle at bedtime will ensure you get a good chunk of sleep, so go to bed early and make use of this time. You would only need to give formula if you do not have enough breast milk for the bedtime bottle or if you have a low milk supply and need to supplement. The aim of the breastfeeding routines is to get one step ahead of your baby's milk demand, which can take weeks. Each feed is a breastfeed which encourages active stimulation as well as expressing to help increase and maintain your supply. This means your baby will be taking all that you are supplying. Your milk supply is personal to you and you may not be able to achieve a milk supply to satisfy your baby's appetite which leaves two options: feeding every 2–3 hours day and night or using expressed breast milk or formula to supplement.

So, giving formula to supplement will not lower your supply if you keep up with the advice in the routines and not replace a breastfeed with formula.

Will breastfeeding for an hour stretch my baby's stomach? I've heard that babies get all the milk they need in the first 5-10 minutes

Firstly, newborns are unable to suck efficiently and take longer to drink their milk than established babies of three months onwards. They need to break regularly to wind and need help staying focused. As your baby grows, her stomach and suck strengthen, she becomes self-winding, and will be able to empty both breasts much more quickly. During the establishing newborn stage your breasts need to build a supply and your flow may not be continuous, but stop-and-start, meaning it takes longer for your baby to feed, so it's important for both you and your baby to allow an hour to make sure she is well-fed and winded in that time – it is not an hour of continuous feeding.

Your milk will thin over the course of the first three months and the flow of milk will speed up from dripping to spraying, so your feeding times will decrease to 30 minutes, or less if your milk is fast-flowing. Feeding a newborn baby for as little as 10 minutes means she will only be getting the thirst-quenching foremilk but not the satisfying and thicker hindmilk and so she will be hungry again very quickly and not be able to go 3–4 hours between feeds. Yes, your baby has a tiny tummy but she will take what will look like a tiny amount of milk to start with and increase this gradually over the weeks as she and her stomach grow. I have also found that the size of the baby doesn't always determine the quantity of milk she takes. Caring for twins over the last 20 years, I often find the smaller twin drinks a larger quantity of milk at each feed as her appetite increases as she is growing to catch up. The rate of growth will determine your baby's appetite.

Towards the end of playtime my baby starts grizzling and roots around when I pick her up. Is she hungry?

It's most likely that your baby is tired, especially if playtime was calm and happy. Babies will root, as if looking for milk, not only when they're hungry but also when they're tired, windy or cross – they want the comfort of sucking rather than the milk. The best thing to do is to give your baby a cuddle to calm her and then put her to bed. However, if she won't settle, it is possible that she is a bit hungry – try increasing her milk intake at each feed and swaddle her for her naps.

When is 'Daddy time' in the routine if I'm breastfeeding?

With most of the families I help, when breastfeeding and teaching both parents my routine and feeding skills, dads take over the bath and bedtime bottle-feed. It's a great time for Dad to have his own quality time of day with his new baby to bond and get involved. Also, having skin-on-skin naps, being chief pram pusher, winder and nappy changer, and maybe even head chef, can be helpful when Mum's days are absorbed by feeding and winding.

Of course, if you are bottle-feeding the routine can be shared equally. It's important to be consistent for the routine to work so keep a baby diary so you can both keep track of what is going on.

Vomiting, Sickness and Posseting

My newborn regularly vomits during the bedtime bottle after the bath

This is a very sensitive time of day as your baby will be feeling tired as he approaches bedtime. The pre-bath feed is essentially there to help make bath time calm and happy. This, of course, can take weeks during the establishing newborn stage. Make sure your baby's pre-bath feed is capped at 60ml (2oz) or 10–15 minutes each side if you're breastfeeding and reduce this time if you think your baby is getting too much milk in this half-hour feed, which is common from Weeks 4–6. Don't be tempted to increase your baby's milk intake at the pre-bath feed as taking too much milk and then sloshing around in the bath will cause vomiting on the post-bath bottle-feed, as well as discouraging the effects of the bedtime bottle and sleeping through the night. Though the majority of mothers have a very low milk supply by 6pm, what they do have may let down quickly. A fast-flowing breast can easily let down over 60ml (2oz) in just five minutes. Reduce the pre-bath bottle to 45ml (1½oz) or five minutes each side until the post-bath feed becomes less problematic.

The post-bath bottle-feed is the largest of all the day feeds and it is important to keep your baby awake and winded well. If you rush this feed, he may take too much milk too quickly and it can cause vomiting. If your baby is a speedy feeder then wind him every 15ml (½oz) instead of 30ml (1oz) to slow the feed down. Another option that works well is to give two-thirds of the bottle steadily with wind breaks and then have a 10-minute break. Make sure you wind your baby and get burps up before stopping for this break. You might want to put your baby somewhere slightly elevated but not too cosy that he falls asleep, like a baby chair or propped slightly at an angle. After the 10-minute break, wind your baby again so you are effectively double-winding him. Too much wind or air which builds while drinking and digesting can cause vomiting. This is not due to overfeeding but simply due to trapped air.

Even babies who have a steady speed of feeding and who have winded beautifully throughout the feed, may need to be winded at 15ml (½oz) intervals for the last 60ml (2oz) as wind is created while digesting and can build up throughout the feed.

Make sure your baby is awake until you put him to bed in order to get the last burp up. For some babies, not getting this last burp up isn't a problem, but more sensitive types may end up vomiting within an hour of going to bed.

If your baby is drinking slowly and falling asleep towards the end of the bottle, and is not actively sucking and swallowing, this sleepy feeding can also cause vomiting. Try keeping him awake and giving a 5–10-minute break to revive him – on the floor (on a muslin) with toys, followed by a nappy change – and then continue with the bottle.

Make sure you have the right size teat and shape for your baby's mouth. A newborn will need a size one teat. If the teat doesn't fit properly in your baby's mouth and lets air in around the corners of his mouth it will be letting in air while he is sucking, creating more gas and increasing the need for winding.

Your baby's milk temperature also needs to be warm. Giving your baby cold milk or milk that has cooled throughout the feed may cause him to gag and be sick and become disinterested in feeding. Warm milk is more appealing for a newborn and is easier to drink and digest. A baby becomes less sensitive to milk temperature at around three months.

Any vomiting which you think is over 30ml (1oz) will need to be re-fed. Your baby has not been sick because he is ill but simply due to wind and digestion (see page 11 for more on this).

If you are giving breast milk throughout the day and night, but giving formula at the bedtime bottle, try swapping this feed for expressed breast milk to see if it's a formula issue. If it is, another option is to try a lactose-free formula and seeing if that makes a difference.

HANDLING AND FEEDING POSITIONS

Your handling and feeding positions could be causing your baby to vomit. At this sensitive time of day, a combination of the feed being the largest of all day feeds and the bath, which is essential to the success of the routine, means you will need to handle your newborn with care, keeping him in a straight position and well-supported while he is feeding. A baby with no stomach muscles and ability to hold his own head will slump naturally. A head that is hung and slumped over, puts pressure on the tummy, which is more likely to make him sick. If you were carried around in a slumped position or laid on your tummy after a meal, you would feel sick too! Keep your baby's back and head held in a straight line over your shoulder, with his back and head fully supported, while carrying him around and feeding.

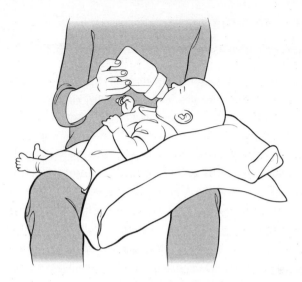

Ideal position for bottle-feeding

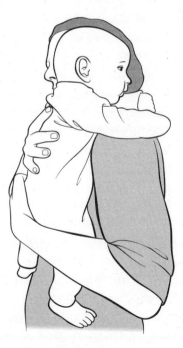

Winding your baby over the shoulder (also the best position for
calming your baby)

Routine Flexibility

How do I fit a routine around my other children?

Establishing a routine around other siblings with different routines can be challenging. Everyone in the family needs to adjust slightly to make room for your new arrival and help establish a routine that eventually is in tune with your other children. This takes weeks, but only weeks, which is a long time in the development of a newborn but only a short time for your other children. The attitude that your newborn needs to fit into your already established lives leaves little room for meeting your baby's needs and helping her sleep well at night. Work out a routine where all your children get the attention they need by firstly looking at the most important time of day: bedtime. Delaying your children's bedtime until after you have put your new baby to bed means siblings will not feel rushed and parents deprived at this important time of day. Adjust the tea or dinner time so it allows you to bath siblings before you start your baby's pre-bath feed or, if you are giving a 60ml (2oz) bottle for the pre-bath feed, tea and bath could be at the same time, but only if your children are old enough to bathe unaided and unattended. Don't be tempted to skip your baby's bath – this is the routine's fourth awake period and helps your newborn recognise that her bottle and bedtime are coming. You will need to focus on your baby's post-bath bottle as this is key to longer sleep periods at night. Your older children could be having reading downtime in their rooms while you are finishing up with your new baby. Alternatively, if both parents are around for bedtime, one parent can focus on the baby while the other spends time with the siblings.

If you are rushed in the mornings with helping everyone else start their day, then wake your baby up for a 6/6.30am start so you can focus and feed her before the rest of the house wakes up. To achieve a full night's sleep you will need to make sure your baby has enough milk and awake time during the day, so if your feed periods clash with school runs then maybe ask for help from friends and family temporarily until your newborn is established and is able to stay awake in motion. This is a short time in your family's life and is well worth investing in. Look at the various feeding routine timings to see how you can fit in your baby's feeds and awake times to allow for digestion and structured play, even if some of the playtime runs short.

Your bedtime routine is the most important as this will be your baby's trickiest time of day and focus is needed to increase the bedtime bottle and keep her awake for this feed in order for her to sleep later through the night.

Can I feed my newborn out and about on the routine?

Yes, but you will need to think ahead. You need to be able to focus on your baby's feed and winding so somewhere like a café is not an ideal environment as it's loud and often hot. A newborn still at the establishing stage will not generally feed herself until she is full, and she is unable to self-wind. She also finds it hard to stay awake while she is digesting her feed. Your baby needs your help and encouragement for the feeds to be successful and to sleep through the night. The more you put in at this stage, the more you will get back sleep-wise. Choose a quiet, cool place to feed your baby where you can stay long enough for the two-hour feed period, such as a friend's house where, if you lose focus, you can pop to another room to get back on track. Travel to your feeding destination during your baby's nap, give her her feed and awake time at your destination and then travel back over the next nap. Newborns are unable to stay awake in motion.

If a full night's sleep is your objective, successful feeding, awake time and naps are key, as well as being consistent with all areas of the routine. If you follow the routine partially you will only get partial results. Once you are established and reach the baby stage from three months onwards, your baby will be able to stay awake during motion, can stay awake in loud, heated cafés, and life suddenly becomes less restricted and free with your baby, who by now sleeps 12 hours through the night.

If my baby wakes before the next feed is due, what do I do?

This is a process of elimination:

- Check your baby is feeding until she is full at each daytime feed and offer her a top-up to see if that makes a difference to the time she wakes.
- Try increasing her overall milk intake and check that she is actively feeding and not snoozing during feeds.
- If you are breastfeeding, make sure your milk supply meets your baby's demand and your diet is wind-free as well as nutritionally dense. Eat between feeds and do not diet.
- Wind your baby thoroughly during and after feeds and allow enough awake time at each day feed period.
- Gradually increase your baby's awake time until she reaches two hours at each feed period.

Keep a baby diary so you can keep track of progress, but also so you can look back to see if a pattern is forming which will help you work out if you are misjudging one of the above on your checklist.

If your baby is still waking early, say 30 minutes before a feed, is hungry and not yet at the stage where she is happy to wait, simply bring the feed forward and adjust your feed timings for the rest of the day. (See below for alternative routine feed timings.)

If she is waking up to an hour before the feed is due, try swaddling her for her day naps, or just the nap that is obviously unsettled, and use the 'shush and hold' technique to resettle her (see page 205). If that doesn't work then cuddle her, kept in her swaddle, or whisk her out quickly in the pram, tucking her in tightly around the shoulders.

How do I change the routine feed times depending on when my baby wakes?

If your baby wakes before 7am or wakes early for the mid-morning feed, below is an alternative feeding schedule to follow. Awake time is timed from the start of the feed for up to two hours which does not include the 10–15-minute wake-up period.

- 6am, 10am, 2pm, 6pm pre-bath feed, 6.30pm bath, 6.45pm bottle, 7.30/8pm bed
- 6.30am, 10/10.30am, 2/2.30pm, 6pm pre-bath feed, 6.30pm bath, 6.45pm bottle, 7.30/8pm bed
- 7am, 10.30/11am, 2.30pm, 6pm pre-bath feed, 6.30pm bath, 6.45pm bottle, 7.30/8pm bed
- 7/7.30am, 11am, 2.30/3pm, 6pm pre-bath feed, 6.30pm bath, 6.45pm bottle, 7.30/8pm bed
- 7.30am, 11.30am, 3pm, 6pm pre-bath feed, 6.30pm bath, 6.45pm bottle, 7.30/8pm bed

I'm using a dummy. How do I get rid of it?

As you know, I'm not a fan of using a dummy unless you are using it temporarily with twins in the last stages of helping them sleep through the night (see page 142). Dummies teach the wrong association with sucking and feeding, encourage comfort sucking, create wind and make digestive issues worse, not to mention introducing settling problems.

A newborn does not naturally suck for comfort. This only starts to happen after three months when teething starts and your baby begins to have control over her hands and is able to put her hands to her mouth and use them as a chew toy. If your baby is comforted by a dummy during the newborn stage, it's likely you have not met all your baby's needs or encouraged self-settling. With any issue, trying to work out your baby's needs is a process of elimination so make sure you are on top of her milk intake and that she is actively sucking and not sleeping during feeds, she is winded thoroughly and has enough awake time.

IF YOU ARE USING A DUMMY FOR SETTLING ...

If your baby won't settle for her daytime naps or at night without a dummy, firstly make sure you are feeding her until she is full at each feed and you are winding her every 30ml (1oz) or every 5–10 minutes on the breast. Offer a top-up after the breastfeed to make sure your baby is full and your issue is not hunger-related. Extend your baby's awake time until she is reaching two hours at each feed period. Swaddle your baby for her daytime naps and for the night and tuck her in tightly so she feels secure and cuddled, and is able to settle without the dummy.

If she is waking at night, try not to react straight away and use the two-minute rule (see page 176). Babies wake frequently in the night and if your baby is sleeping in your room you may find it hard to wait through two minutes of proper crying, perhaps jumping to each squeak and grizzle. A baby sleeping in your bedroom will be more disturbed at night as she can hear your snores, turning in bed or getting up for the loo. If she is not waking due to hunger but as a habit, try the 'shush and hold' technique (see page 205).

Breaking a dummy habit at night can be tricky as babies become reliant on it to resettle. It is often less stimulating than any other resettling technique as you can quickly pop the dummy in rather than 'shush and hold', which can stimulate your baby awake once she becomes more aware at around Weeks 6–8 and is used to sucking for comfort. Your day routine determines your nights so using other settling techniques, such as encouraging self-settling during the day, having calm down time before naps, waiting two minutes between shush and hold to calm your baby, swaddling and creating a positive sleep environment, will have a positive knock-on effect on settling your baby at night (see Chapter Thirteen for more on this). Consistency is key if you want a technique to work: going cold turkey on the dummy use during the day, only to give in and use a dummy at 3am, will set you back to square one.

IF YOU ARE USING A DUMMY TO DELAY FEEDS ...

If you are using a dummy to delay a day feed, stop using the dummy and feed your baby instead. There is no point using a dummy to settle your baby as feeding will have the same result. Hunger is obviously the cause of waking so focus on increasing your baby's overall milk intake so she is satisfied between feeds. Sorting out your day routine will help phase out night waking.

IF YOU ARE USING A DUMMY TO CALM YOUR BABY BEFORE AND AFTER FEEDS ...

Newborns have a strong fight-or-flight instinct and will generally scream or cry until they are fed. It takes weeks for your baby to understand she won't starve and that food is coming. Walk around with your baby over your shoulder to calm her, pat and shush her, or simply feed her early if she can't wait.

Using a dummy after a feed would indicate that your baby is still hungry or still has wind. Try topping her up with a bottle, increasing your milk supply, increasing her overall day feeds and winding frequently.

If you are already in a dummy habit and your baby is over eight weeks old, putting my routine into practice will mean the only reason your baby will want the dummy will be out of habit. Start weaning her off the dummy during the day, using distraction instead of a dummy to calm her during playtime. At nap times use other settling techniques, such as shush and hold until calm and waiting two minutes before trying again, at least 3–4 times before giving the dummy. If you do use the dummy to settle your baby then wait until she is calm and take the dummy out of her mouth before leaving the room so she is not left sleeping with it. Be consistent in trying other options, such as the settling techniques suggested on page 204 or taking your baby out in the pram. Even delaying the dummy use will help your baby understand it's not an immediate comforter or sleep aid. You could go cold turkey and throw the dummy away to stop you giving in at 4am which is, of course, often a more painful approach for all parties, but is a quicker way to resolve dummy dependency.

I do understand that sometimes it's easier to use a prop, like a dummy, for a peaceful night's sleep and for some quiet time during the day when you are frazzled and not sure how to read your baby, but, ultimately, this will be a longer route in your quest for a full night's sleep. From three months of age you will find that your baby starts chewing and sucking on her hands and anything she is able to hold. By this time the startle reflex has calmed so she is no longer woken by jumping arms and legs and is able to sleep peacefully without a swaddle. She may even start sucking a thumb or finger. You might think a dummy is perfect as you can throw it away when you attempt to break the sucking habit, unlike a thumb or finger, but your baby will be unable to pick up a dummy and pop it back in her mouth until she is much older so the dummy falling out will cause night waking, often more so than during the newborn stage of night feeds.

Awake Time and Naps
My four-week-old will only sleep for 30 minutes during his afternoon nap

The more solidly your baby sleeps during the night, the less sleep he needs during the day. The first nap to be impacted by this is generally the afternoon nap, and this usually starts to be affected anywhere from six weeks. When this happens adjust your feed times to: 7am, 11am, 3pm, 6pm pre-bath feed, 6.30pm bath, 6.45pm bottle, 7.30pm bed. This leaves a shorter gap between the afternoon and pre-bath feeds and a shorter nap period of 45 minutes between 5pm and 5.45pm. If your baby sleeps for 20–30 minutes of this time, this should be enough to see him through until bedtime.

When breastfeeding, your milk supply depletes throughout the day and, for some mothers, it dramatically depletes by the afternoon feed. It could be that your baby is not getting enough milk to sleep well at the afternoon nap. Reduce your afternoon breastfeed to 45–50 minutes and use the last 10–15 minutes of the feed to top up with a bottle of expressed breast milk and see if your baby is eager to take the extra milk. Test your milk supply by expressing straight after the afternoon feed to see what's left and whether you have run out of milk. You can also test your supply by expressing the afternoon feed, 30 minutes before the feed time, to check what you're producing. If these two tests confirm you have a low milk supply, introduce a top-up at the afternoon feed and look to increase your supply by resting during the lunchtime nap, eating between feeds and drinking plenty of water (see page 32 for more on this). If you are running around and generally being busy this will work against your supply. You will either need to slow down or introduce top-ups as a regular part of your routine and perhaps look to mix feed (Chapter Six). You might otherwise find that your little one is reluctant to phase out his night feeds.

Having enough awake time during the day will have an impact on how well your baby sleeps during his naps. Increase your baby's awake time to two hours at each feed period if you have not reached this already. If you are at the two-hour mark for each awake period, increase all awake time to 2¼ hours. Do not go over this time as your baby needs good-quality naps to be able to feed and stay awake at the right times of day.

Stretching the morning awake time to longer than advised can also mean your baby is unable to stay awake during the afternoon awake time and then wakes early before the pre-bath feed.

My baby is wakeful in the morning and sleeps all afternoon and then wakes too early for the pre-bath feed

Structuring your baby's awake time evenly will encourage him to feed well at each feed period and get into the routine of feeding, awake/playtime and then nap time. Some babies are sprightlier in the mornings, having slept well at night, but having too long awake time in the mornings interferes with their afternoon feeds and playtime. You may think it a positive thing if your baby can stay awake happily playing in excess of two hours after his morning feed, only to find he is unable to stay awake and feed properly for the mid-morning or afternoon feeds. During the first four weeks of life, while your newborn is waking up to the world, the length of time he is able to stay awake can vary, with some babies taking weeks to be able to stay awake for all of their awake and play periods. It's common for a newborn under four weeks old to only manage two out of three awake periods. If you allow your baby to stay awake for longer than two hours in the morning then he will struggle with the rest of the day. Cap his awake time to 1½–1¾ hours until he is able to stay awake for all three awake periods and then look to increase all awake periods to two hours.

Not having awake time in the afternoon means your baby is bound to wake early and disrupt the intended routine. He may need a little more encouragement to wake for playtime and feeds in the afternoon. A cool water nappy change or even a strip wash will help to revive him.

If your baby wakes often in the night, this alone will have an impact on his wakefulness during the day. The more wake-ups at night the sleepier he will be during the day. The effort you put into your day routine will turn this around as it all boils down to his daily milk intake and awake time.

Make sure you are creating the right environment for your baby to be able to stay awake during feeds and playtime. Going out and about, pram pushing, café feeding, group meetings and baby clubs are not going to encourage wakefulness. Your baby is learning the difference between night and day and is extremely sensitive to sound, heat and light and is easily cuddled and lulled to sleep by the environment (see page 188). If you are going out, arrange to do so during your baby's nap time and then find somewhere cool and quiet to focus on his feeds and awake time.

If your baby is still struggling to wake for the afternoon playtime and wakes early for the pre-bath feed, try the 'shush and hold' technique (page 205). If this doesn't work, simply cuddle him back to sleep until his waking time is due or start the evening bedtime routine early. You may need to wait a few weeks while he grows and wakes up a bit more to the world around him before he is able to stay awake for longer periods. Lastly, make sure you set up the right environment to nap, in his own room, swaddled and tucked into bed (see Chapter Thirteen).

I'm struggling to keep my newborn awake for playtime

Keeping your baby awake while feeding will help and encourage awake time while he digests his milk. Babies are naturally sleepy after feeds, as their bodies heat up while feeding and digesting. Keep your baby cool for playtime, as you would during feeds, and don't rush to put his clothes back on. If the room temperature is between 19°C and 20°C, this is certainly warm enough to play in just a short-sleeved bodysuit with his arms and legs left bare. Summer babies in my care are rarely in a sleepsuit or Babygro that cover their arms and legs during the day, much to the upset of grandparents who still think you need to keep newborns dressed up in lots of layers, hats and blankets! Overheating with a full and often windy tummy will result in your newborn falling asleep after his feeds. A newborn is unable to stay awake while in motion or outside, so make sure your feeds and awake times are indoors, in a calm and quiet environment.

Saving a nappy change until after a feed will also help to revive your baby. If this doesn't work, you could try a strip wash on the changing table, with tepid water in the winter months and cool water in the summer months. Your baby is more likely to stay awake if you put him down to play on a play mat instead of cuddling or holding him on your lap. Engage him with black-and-white pictures and toys or, if he is a little older and is able to track movement (from eight weeks old), place him somewhere he can see you and watch you moving around the room. Using squeaky sound toys will also help as your baby finds high-pitched noises stimulating.

Don't worry if you are unable to keep your baby awake for as long as recommended in my routines. Try to stretch the playtime out by around 10 minutes at a time. Encouraging the awake time is all you can do. If your baby really won't wake up then put him to bed in a swaddle as it will help keep him sleeping until the next feed. Having no awake time after a feed means you run the risk of having a disturbed nap or your baby waking too early for the next feed period. As your baby grows he will have days where he can stay awake easily and others where he will struggle. Be consistent in your attempts to wake him at each feed for playtime and soon the routine will click into place, and no doubt you will move on to some other challenge! The more your baby sleeps at night, the more wakeful your days will be.

If your baby is not winded effectively during the feed, a build-up of gas can make him feel bloated and sleepy. Your newborn will also need to be winded during playtime while digesting milk to help keep him awake.

My eight-week-old is sleeping through the night but wakes often during his daytime naps

Check how much milk your baby is taking and whether he has had enough awake time. If he is not getting enough milk at each feed, none of the settling or routine changes will work to resolve his disturbed naps. Express a feed to see how much milk you are producing and give a bottle instead. Make sure you express for long enough and stop–start the stimulating setting to give variations on speed and suction. If bottle-feeding, look to increase each day feed by 30ml (1oz) at a time until the problem is solved. A baby under three months of age should be able to sleep through the night for 10–12 hours and have 3–4 hours' nap time.

My routine encourages a full night's sleep which is reached much earlier than commonly thought possible. The trade-off is that less sleep or less solid sleep is needed during the day. This is, of course, the right way round but often a newborn is unable to stay awake longer than 2–2¼ hours until he reaches three months onwards. Usually it's the afternoon nap which is the first to become unsettled and phased out. If this is the case then move your afternoon feed to 3pm (adjusting all other previous day feeds). This leaves 45 minutes for an afternoon nap which, if only slept for 30 minutes, should be enough for an active successful bottle and bedtime routine. If the morning nap is unsettled or your baby wakes early for the mid-morning feed, until he is able to wait happily for feeds extend his awake time to 2¼ hours at each feed period. This should be timed from the start of a feed, not including the 10–15-minute waking time.

Create the right environment for your baby's naps and put him down to sleep in a cot, Moses basket or pram. If you are pushing your baby out in a pram for every nap this will make for settling issues as he is taught to sleep in motion. Find a balance so at least one nap – the lunchtime nap being the most ideal – is in his own room (see Chapter Thirteen).

If your baby is waking early for feeds, leave him for two minutes to see if he resettles but, if waking within 30 minutes of the normal waking time, it's unlikely for a newborn to resettle as hunger will be setting in. Adjust the routine to feed your baby 15 minutes early or distract him with a cuddle until the usual feed time. If he is waking, say, within an hour of his feed time, then shush and hold him to try and resettle him (see page 205). Repeat as necessary with two-minute intervals so you are not jumping to his every shout out. Often babies will wake briefly and resettle themselves. As a last resort, take him out in the pram or give him a cuddle. If you are no longer swaddling during daytime naps, reintroduce the swaddle which will help your baby sleep for longer.

The amount of sleep your newborn or baby needs is personal to him and, once he is sleeping through the night, the length of sleep needed during the day can vary dramatically, with some babies dropping a nap by Week 6 while others will still have three naps at six months. Of all the daytime naps, the lunchtime/midday nap is the most beneficial and will be the last nap your baby drops – this nap can continue until he is three years old. Having a long nap over the lunchtime period can be encouraged by limiting your baby's morning nap, but this can only be done once your baby is able to happily play and wait for feeds. This is usually from Weeks 8–10 onwards. Extend your baby's morning awake time and cut his morning nap by 15 minutes at a time until the lunchtime nap has become settled.

My baby cries every time I try and put him down to play

Firstly check that your baby is full and winded well, and offer him more milk if you think he is still hungry. If he takes the extra milk easily, he is still hungry and will not be happy to play until he is full.

The first part of the awake time – straight after a feed – is the happiest time for your baby to play by himself. A baby with a full tummy who is winded well should be happy to play unless, of course, he is used to being picked up on every cry out or grizzle and walked around all day, and therefore unable to play contentedly by himself. This is very common as a newborn becomes more aware from Week 4. Your baby will quickly learn that the best place to be is with you, and over the weeks will become bored of his surroundings. To combat this try toy rotation or changing the black-and-white picture you are using. Maybe your baby is starting to track and follow and now needs something more interactive? (See page 192 for more on this.)

Instead of reacting and picking him up straight away, try the two-minute rule, using your voice to distract him and holding his feet firmly. By holding his feet, your baby will feel your touch and recognise that you are there which usually calms and makes a newborn feel secure. When the startle reflex kicks in, from Weeks 3–6, his jerky limb movements can be unsettling. Keep going with the foot-hold technique while it works until you need to pick him up. Once you have picked your baby up have some one-on-one time with him. Chat, talk and play for 10 minutes or so before putting him down to play again and entertain himself. Find a balance between a cuddle and bonding, and building your baby's confidence; constant picking up and down is confusing for a baby and won't have a settling effect, but may upset him more. Your newborn will only be happy to play and look around on a play mat, looking at black-and-white pictures, when he has been fed and is well rested. He will not be happy to play before a feed in the first 6–8 weeks or if he is tired.

Towards the end of your newborn's playtime he may get grumpy as he starts to become tired. During the last half an hour of the playtime, he has digested his milk enough to have tummy time or chat time with you to distract him until he needs to nap.

You may also need to check for wind a few times during playtime while he is still digesting his milk, which can cause a few grizzles until he has burped.

My baby cries when I try and put him down for a nap

Has your baby had happy and content playtime? If the answer is yes then his cries are unlikely to be due to hunger or not having had enough awake time. If he has not reached the two-hour awake target then gradually extend his awake time until he reaches the recommended two hours. If he is unsettled and unhappy during playtime you will need to look at his feeds and milk intake.

Babies often cry before they fall asleep and, if left for a few minutes, will settle themselves. The older and more aware a baby gets, the more he needs a 10–15-minute cuddle to calm down before bed. It's unfair to expect a baby to go straight from the play mat to bed.

If you are still in the first eight weeks, use a swaddle to help settle your baby as most young babies find it hard to settle with their arms exposed. If your baby is older than eight weeks and you are not using a swaddle, always make sure you tuck him tightly into his Moses basket, pram or cot (see Chapter Thirteen). Babies like to feel secure to drift off to sleep.

Are you carrying your baby around all day? Could he be crying because he is not used to being put down? Encouraging playtime by himself without the need to be cuddled and carried will build your baby's confidence to settle to play and sleep by himself. A baby who is constantly picked up and down and not left to settle unaided will not be able to self-settle. Instead of picking your baby up, wait two minutes then use the 'shush and hold' technique (see page 205). Find a balance between a cuddle and bonding time, and building your baby's confidence. Your newborn will only be happy to play and look around on a play mat, looking at black-and-white pictures, when he has been fed and is well rested.

My baby won't settle to bed at 7.30pm

This is an unlikely scenario on my routine, especially during the first six weeks, as it's more of a problem keeping your baby awake long enough to take the bedtime bottle. Still, not settling to bed is not unheard of and usually occurs with babies of a certain temperament – those who are quite vocal about what they do and don't like! If your routine is working well during the day and your baby is feeding well, is happy to stay awake during playtime and is able to settle to sleep during the day, it's likely to be an issue surrounding the bedtime routine.

This is the only time of day your baby will go to sleep on a full tummy. Make sure he wakes to burp/wind before settling to sleep and also try keeping him awake for 5–10 minutes after the feed to digest and burp a second time before putting him to bed. It's important that your baby is fully winded and comfortable before being put to bed otherwise wind could be the culprit that is stopping him settling well.

If you have spent most of the post-bath bottle waking your baby constantly to take his milk and wind, he may find it hard to settle once he is eventually finished. Once he is put to bed and the room is dark and quiet, he may notice the environment change and wake up again. Swaddle and cuddle him until he is calm and check for more wind over your shoulder.

Has your baby fallen asleep prematurely and not taken enough milk? Are you finding it hard to increase his milk intake at this time of day? Try reducing his pre-bath milk intake, keep his bath cool and maybe temporarily start the bottle 15 minutes earlier. Offer more milk after checking for wind and see if he has suddenly decided he is still hungry.

This is the only time of day you would not use the two-minute rule if your baby has problems settling. Being the only time he is put to bed on a full tummy it's important you do react immediately, pick him up and wind him over your shoulder. Check that the swaddle is tight and cuddle him until he is calm, then gently put him back to bed and tuck him in. If he still won't settle, offer him another 30–60ml (1–2oz) of milk.

A newborn can often seem fickle. They look full and disinterested in milk only to cry for a feed 20 minutes later. These babies of a certain temperament often do things in their own time and I think it is a sign of a strong personality which will hold them in good stead as adults. To name one baby who stands out in the last 20 years: Poppy!

My newborn is almost sleeping through the night but wakes at 4am every morning!

I often have a newborn who will wake on the dot every night, not for hunger but out of habit. It's sometimes easier to tackle night waking when a baby is randomly waking and bouncing around at any hour of the night. If you are still feeding your baby at 4am try gradually reducing the amount of milk he is having by 60–90ml (2–3oz) maximum or 5–15 minutes on one breast. Keep your baby swaddled to feed (re-swaddle before feeding if it has come loose) and keep the room as dark as possible. The idea is to phase this feed out gradually with time on the breast or quantity from a bottle, which will discourage waking.

If you are not offering milk at 4am, try the two-minute rule (page 176) then shush and hold until your baby is calm, and repeat, trying not to pick him up. If you do pick your baby up then don't leave the room, cuddle him back to sleep, sat or lying down. Do not be tempted to walk around or rock your baby which will effectively overstimulate him. If you are calm your baby will eventually calm down, so keep to the same position, hold him tightly and pat him back to sleep.

Look to increase your baby's overall daily milk intake and make sure all his awake periods are up to two hours. Make sure you are not putting your baby to bed too early. Extend his bedtime to 7.30/8pm and wake him for the morning feed by 6.45am every morning, regardless of your night's sleep, to encourage him to sleep later than 4am. Once he starts to move past this time, keep the changes until he sleeps through to 6am or 7am. You could also temporarily change your routine to four-hourly, with a 6am start, which will give your baby a longer daytime until he starts to sleep later again through the night.

Another trick which you could try if nothing else works is to set your alarm and wake him at random times between 2am and 3.30am to break the 4am habitual waking.

What's the best calming position for a baby?

To soothe and calm a crying baby the best place is the shoulder hold, or 'top spot' as I like to call it. Holding your baby tightly against your chest with his head over your shoulder means you can shush him to calm him as his face is next to yours. Ideally keep still and, with calm, deep breathing, pat your baby's back and bottom. As a last resort, walk around, but don't change the hold position. Babies respond to confidence and feeling secure, which is why the swaddle works so well. Cradling your baby in your arms is a feeding position and often causes frustration and confusion. Constant rocking and changing of positions also causes confusion and more stress as you are not giving off calm and confident vibes. See page 205 for more advice on calming your baby.

My newborn likes to sleep with his hands out. Can I leave the swaddling out of my routine?

Yes you can, but you may not get the result of sleeping through the night as quickly as if your baby was swaddled. Newborns will be disturbed by the startle reflex which will encourage night waking. They will also be disturbed and woken by your noises if they are sleeping in your bedroom. Swaddled babies will sleep for longer as they feel secure and cuddled. The swaddle is another key factor to how long your baby will sleep during the newborn stage, as it encourages night sleeping and helps a baby to recognise the difference between night and day.

Often babies will not like the process of being swaddled, much as they don't like a bath, nappy change or getting dressed, but once they are swaddled and sleeping they will sleep more peacefully and soon learn that being swaddled means it's time for bed and the simple process of swaddling will calm them down.

Try swaddling at night only, so you get the best of both worlds. If you are starting my routine from Week 8 and your baby has started chewing his hands, you could half swaddle with the top arm out as a compromise, but certainly during the first six weeks full swaddle at night to gain the benefits of longer sleep periods at night.

My newborn is sleeping through until 5am – the 'no feed zone' – but I'm unable to get him back to sleep or settle until 6am

Settling your baby back to sleep at this time is often a challenge as he will have already slept for around nine hours or more. The key is for as little stimulation as possible. Your first step should be to leave two minutes longer for him to stop crying, then use the shush and hold technique without taking him out of his bed, making sure he is still wrapped tightly in his swaddle. Repeat this technique while it works, even if that is for just five minutes. The next step is to pick your baby up and hold him tightly on your chest (cover any bare skin with a muslin or top) and go back to bed or sit in a chair in his room. Pat his bottom in a rhythmic, soothing – not a frantic – way and shush. Once he is calm, breathe deeply to relax yourself and your baby. Keep your baby in the same position on your chest. If this still doesn't work to settle him, then let him suck on your finger. This technique has never failed me, but I will only ever use it for the 5am 'no feed' hour.

Make sure that, whichever room you are resettling your baby in, it is dark and no light is streaming in from outside, which is another reason for waking at this time of the morning. If you have a summer baby, make sure to install blackout blinds to keep the room dark until you need him to wake at 7am. Do not change your baby's nappy or talk and engage his brain which will, of course, stimulate him awake.

Implementing a Routine at a Later Stage

My baby is already six weeks old and not on a routine. How do I start?

Here is a guide to implementing structure. First, decide on a feeding routine that suits your lifestyle. Below are five feeding timing options which also show you how you can adapt and change your routine on a daily basis if your baby wakes early or is unable to reach the next day feed and is too hungry to wait. You may also have other children you need to work around and consider.

1. 6am, 10am, 2pm, 6pm pre-bath feed, 6.30pm bath, 6.45pm bottle, 7.30/8pm bed
2. 6.30am, 10/10.30am, 2/2.30pm, 6pm pre-bath feed, 6.30pm bath, 6.45pm bottle, 7.30/8pm bed
3. 7am, 10.30/11am, 2.30pm, 6pm pre-bath feed, 6.30pm bath, 6.45pm bottle, 7.30/8pm bed
4. 7/7.30am, 11am, 2.30/3pm, 6pm pre-bath feed, 6.30pm bath, 6.45pm bottle, 7.30/8pm bed
5. 7.30am, 11.30am, 3pm, 6pm pre-bath feed, 6.30pm bath, 6.45pm bottle, 7.30/8pm bed

Before you are able to move on to one of these feeding routines, gradually space out the daytime feeds from on-demand feeding to three-hourly feeds during the day and leave your baby to wake of her own accord at night. Increase her intake of milk at each day feed by extending the time on each breast and allowing an hour for feeds during the day and 30 minutes for night feeds. Cap the night bottles at 120ml (4oz) per feed and reduce the amount of milk given at any one feed the later your baby wakes at night (see page 64). After a few days of three-hourly feeding and increasing your baby's milk intake you should be able to move on to one of the above feeding routines. Try to keep your baby awake for up to two hours at each daytime feed by having playtime after each feed (the two hours includes the time taken to feed, change her nappy, etc.).

Even if your baby is sleeping well during the day you will need to wake her for feeds, waking her 10–15 minutes before each day feed to give her time to wake up and be ready for the feed. Never let her go for more than four hours between daytime feeds, while there should be at least 4–5 hours between night feeds. Split the bedtime feed with a bath and give a bottle of milk before bed. The pre-bath feed is capped at 10–15 minutes each side, or 60ml (2oz) from the bottle, which includes winding every five minutes. If the bottle is a struggle after the bath, reduce the pre-bath feed. The temperature of the bath water can also make a difference to how well your baby takes her bedtime bottle – 34–35°C maximum is ideal.

Expressing after day feeds will increase your milk supply during the day and, of course, increase your baby's daily milk intake. The routines will not work unless your baby has had enough milk, so getting to know your supply is of the utmost importance. Top up if needed, which will also test to see if your baby is still hungry.

If your baby is bottle-feeding then increase her milk intake by 30ml (1oz) per feed during the day until she is sleeping through the night. Her milk intake will reach between 200ml (7oz) and 260ml (9oz) per feed. The afternoon feed is your least important feed of the day and is generally 30ml (1oz) less than the morning feeds, which helps increase your baby's appetite for the evening bottle, which is usually 30–60ml (1–2oz) more than the morning feeds. Cap your pre-bath feed at 60ml (2oz) which can only increase to 90ml (3oz) once your baby is taking over 240ml (8oz) post-bath.

Introduce a swaddle for night sleeping and daytime naps if you find settling an issue to begin with. Please refer to Chapter One to make sure you are on top of and understand your baby's digestion and how often you need to wind her. An increase of daily milk intake won't be possible unless your baby is wind-free.

I'm on the 7pm–7am routine and my baby slept through the night for the first time last night but woke at 6am. Should I give a short feed at 6am and then again at 7am?

The routine is flexible to the time your baby wakes in the morning so you are able to start your day anywhere from 6am and the feed timings will allow you to put your baby to bed at her usual bedtime. There are various combinations of feed timings on my routine which all end the day at the same time, so you have consistency with your baby's bedtime which means your baby has more chance of sleeping through the night. Start your day at 6am and adjust all the other feeds to a four-hourly feeding routine: 6am, 10am, 2pm, 6pm and 6.45pm. It can take some time before your baby is able to sleep until 7am so let your feeding routine be flexible to her waking time.

If your baby wakes at 5am, this is a 'no feed' hour. Giving even the smallest amount of milk at this time will interfere with her morning feed. Resettle your baby back to sleep by cuddling her (keep her swaddled) or, as a last resort, let her suck on your finger and then start your day at 6am. See page 119 for more advice on this.

My baby slept through the night at four weeks old for two weeks, so why has she now started waking at 4am?

Keeping a diary during the newborn stage will help you keep track of any changes to your baby's routine. As your baby grows, in the first six weeks especially, her intake of milk and awake time will also increase. The routine needs to evolve as she grows so make sure you are keeping up with her appetite and increasing her daily intake of milk, especially at the bedtime bottle. Yes, once she sleeps through the night she has reached her personal magic number of ounces per day for this to happen, but you will need to be consistent with the routine to solidify it and for night sleeping to become habitual.

Your baby may well be sleeping through the night having not yet reached staying awake for two hours at each feed period during the day, so keep encouraging this over the coming weeks. Add an extra 30ml (1oz) in the bedtime bottle for whenever she decides to increase her milk intake. She will be hitting a major growth spurt at six weeks old and will no doubt have an increase of appetite as well as becoming more aware of her surroundings. Make sure there have not been any changes, such as room temperature. If she is too cold, she will wake up. Has she become more active and wriggled out of her swaddle? Is it summer and light is coming through the curtains causing early waking? For whatever reason she has started waking up again, try and resettle her initially without feeding. If you need to feed then give her the shortest feed possible. Keep her swaddled or re-swaddle her so she is secure. Don't change her nappy (unless it is dirty) and feed for five minutes on the breast, just enough to resettle, or 60ml (2oz) if bottle-feeding.

Keep on top of your day routine as this is where you will find the reason for waking. It is common for babies who sleep through the night at such an early age to backtrack slightly.

Twin Solutions

How do I feed my babies at the same time?

Tandem feeding makes easy work of a twin routine and, once you have nailed your technique, it is the most wonderful bonding experience: the angle at which you feed your babies, whether it be breast or bottle, means you have two faces staring up at you and then at each other – a three-way bond. Tandem feeding can be a little challenging to start with and also quite straining on your neck and shoulders. As a twin routine specialist for 20 years I am aware of how important it is to get the perfect position and posture to feed. Focusing on two babies means you cannot take your eyes off your babies and you need to switch your focus every few sucks to make sure they stay active. It's like watching a game of feeding tennis! You need a lot of focus to actively feed just one baby, making sure he is feeding well and not comfort sucking, so, with twins, feed times need to be quiet with no distractions, such as lots of visitors and watching TV. However, an extra pair of hands to help you wind, tickle their feet and warm bottles will make feeds much easier, especially in the early days.

Make sure you are sat with your back straight and arms in a comfortable position to feed. You will be looking down at your babies which, over time, can affect your neck. Having good posture will help with this, but if you do develop neck and shoulder stiffness this can restrict your milk flow when breastfeeding, given the added tension. A microwave wheat bag works well to alleviate tension during and after feeds. When bottle-feeding your babies they can be in a more forward position in front of you rather than at a head-to-breast level.

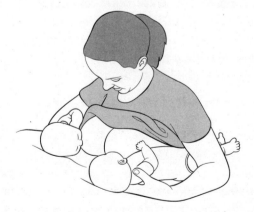

Ideal position for tandem breastfeeding

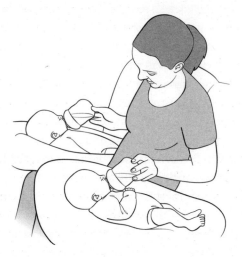

Ideal position for tandem bottle-feeding

Get prepared with the bottles ready to go for the swap over from breast to bottle, have water and snacks for yourself to hand, and the breast pump sterilised and set up ready for action. To tandem feed you will need a sofa and two square pillows or a twin breastfeeding pillow, such as Peanut & Piglet. Latch the most demanding baby or easiest latching baby first, hold him in place with your hand and then latch the second. You may need help to do this until you get used to the positioning and how your babies move. Please see Chapter Ten for more advice on this.

How do I move on from tandem feeding?

As your babies get bigger, they start to move and kick their arms and legs around so it may become increasingly difficult to tandem feed, usually from around 10 weeks of age. Moving on from tandem feeding can be done in stages as tandem feeding gets increasingly hard towards the mid to end of the feed as your babies become full and less enthusiastic or distracted while feeding, making hard work of keeping them both actively feeding and focused. Start the feeds tandem until you are unable to feed them together, then feed singularly for the rest of the feed by swapping each baby at wind breaks.

When tandem feeding on feeding pillows is no longer an option, which can start from around 10–12 weeks of age, you can try using baby chairs to continue tandem feeding with the bottles after the breastfeed. Baby chair feeding isn't recommended until Week 8 when your babies need less help to feed and become more efficient. Alternatively, feed your babies singularly by offering the most enthusiastic twin his milk first, feed for only 5–10 minutes on the breast or 30–60ml (1–2oz) on the bottle each, and then swap babies, swapping every 30–60ml (1–2oz) or 5–10 minutes on the breast until the end of the feed. You will have feeds where one twin will be hungry and efficient and the other sleepy and slow. When this happens, start the feed giving equal amounts, but when the sleepy twin is looking disinterested and won't suck, finish the efficient twin and then focus on the inactive twin once your enthusiastic twin has finished. This technique works well when you have one twin that is not winding and has a stuck air bubble – he can wait and have a break while you are focusing mainly on the active twin, then swap babies again. When you are approaching the end of the feed, keep the twin on a feeding break slightly propped and not lying flat on his back. A baby who has a stuck air bubble and is more than midway through a feed can easily vomit if left too long flat on his back. Lying flat helps move the wind out, but will also bring up milk.

How do I wind while tandem feeding?

It is possible to wind one twin while still feeding the other during a bottle- or breastfeed, but it's an advanced move and easier once your babies have developed their stomach muscles. In the meantime, time the feed to break every 5–10 minutes or when they start to slow down. While bottle-feeding you should break to wind, regardless, every 30ml (1oz). If after 5–10 minutes one twin is active and the other is slowing down, then break them both to wind. Wake them up on a muslin on the floor and wind one at a time then re-latch them both for another five minutes or so. If one twin is active and the other is not after 1–3 minutes, keep the active twin sucking and de-latch the inactive twin and tickle him with your free hand. Towards the end of the feed they will become harder to wake and wind so you may need to feed the last 30–60ml (1–2oz) singularly. If you are feeding one twin at a time, prop the waiting twin on a feeding pillow next to you if he is fully awake. Leaving him flat on the floor on a play mat may cause vomiting, but it is the best place to help bring up wind and wake your baby up. Before continuing to feed, wake and wind before focusing on the twin you are feeding, making sure both babies are awake regardless if they are being fed or having a break.

If you are bottle-feeding but can't tandem feed, give the hungriest baby his milk first until the edge is taken off his appetite and then move to the second and keep swapping. You can use this feeding method once your babies become too old to tandem feed and wake up happy and able to wait for feeds.

How do I stop my newborn twins falling asleep without having a free hand to encourage activity?

Keeping two babies active while feeding means you will need to break more often to wind them and enable them to refocus. Depending on the size of your babies and breasts, with feeding cushions you may be able to latch them on and have them in a position where you do not need to hold them on, giving a free hand to tickle and prompt each baby. But if you do need to hold your babies' heads while they feed and have no free hands then frequent breaking is your only option. Make sure the room is cool and strip your babies to vest bodysuits only to feed. When breastfeeding, use a feeding pillow where possible, like the Peanut & Piglet twin feeding pillow, which is firm so your babies won't be encased by a soft pillow which will make feeding too cosy and soporific. Otherwise use two firm, square bed pillows. When bottle-feeding, hold the bottles further down towards the teat so you can use your fingers to stroke your babies' cheeks. If one baby starts to become inactive, and the other is feeding well, break the inactive twin and tickle him with your free hand until you can break the second twin as he slows down. Wake and wind both babies and then start again.

Index